THE POSTPARTUM CHECK-IN

THE POSTPARTUM CHECK-IN

WHAT'S NORMAL, WHAT'S NOT, AND HOW TO ADVOCATE FOR THE CARE YOU DESERVE

DR. ALEXANDRA MACKILLOP

Revell
a division of Baker Publishing Group
Grand Rapids, Michigan

Published by Revell
a division of Baker Publishing Group
Grand Rapids, Michigan
RevellBooks.com

Printed in the United States of America

Library of Congress Cataloging-in-Publication Data
Names: MacKillop, Alexandra, 1994– author
Title: The postpartum check-in : what's normal, what's not, and how to advocate for the care you deserve / Alexandra MacKillop.
Description: Grand Rapids : Revell, a division of Baker Publishing Group, 2026. | Includes bibliographical references.
Identifiers: LCCN 2026007759 | ISBN 9780800748593 paperback | ISBN 9781493455591 ebook
Subjects: LCSH: Postpartum depression | Postpartum depression—Treatment | Motherhood
Classification: LCC RG852 .M32 2026 | DDC 618.7/6—dc23/eng/20260507
LC record available at https://lccn.loc.gov/2026007759

Cover design by Alecia Sharp

The author is represented by WordServe Literary Group, www.wordserveliterary.com.

Baker Publishing Group publications use paper produced from sustainable forestry practices and postconsumer waste whenever possible.

26 27 28 29 30 31 32 7 6 5 4 3 2 1

To the mom who wonders
if it's just supposed to be this hard

Contents

Dear reader,

It is such a privilege and an honor to have earned your trust, enough for you to look to my words for help at the tender and vulnerable place that is postpartum. My deepest hope is that this book will be a guide and a help to you as you navigate your health during this important transition in your life.

That being said, please know that this book is intended to be used as an educational tool only, with the goal of helping you better understand your body and advocate for yourself in a medical setting. It is not intended to be used as a replacement for healthcare, including diagnosis or treatment from a licensed provider. In other words, it is not intended to diagnose, treat, cure, or prevent any disease. Please always consult with your own doctor before implementing any health-related strategies that you read about in this book or anywhere else.

On the note of patient care, I also want to acknowledge that over the course of this text, I share patient anecdotes to illustrate certain points, make connections, and relate to you as a reader. Please know that while these stories reflect real clinical concerns that are commonplace in my practice, all personal details have been removed and a fictional mannequin created to fill the role of conveying relevant clinical information. The dialogue in this book represents, but is not to be taken as an accurate record of, patient conversation. Rather, I ask you to view it as a reflection of some of the most common and most important experiences shared among many of my patients and among women everywhere. Protecting the privacy of the real-life people who have chosen to entrust me with their health is of utmost importance to me. Thank you for your understanding in this matter.

In health,

Dr. Alexandra
MacKillop, DC

PART 1

What Nobody Told You About "Normal" Postpartum

CHAPTER 1

Being a New Mom Isn't a Disease

One of the earliest pieces of advice I received in my first pregnancy was to keep my schedule light—not just in the early postpartum days but throughout my baby's infancy and even toddlerdom. It made sense, I figured. Parenting would be tiring; I'd be sleep-deprived. I should protect my energy by setting boundaries around my schedule. But I had no idea just how tiring it all would be and how much I'd need to take that advice to heart.

When my son was born, I spent the first several weeks doing little else besides snuggling him. He was so cute and the sleeplessness was so hard that cuddling seemed like the perfect way to fill time between feedings. After all, the other things that I needed to do, like use the bathroom and shower, required so many extra steps that there really wasn't much time or energy for anything else. Trips to the pediatrician felt like a whole-day affair, what with packing the diaper bag, doing multiple feedings in the car, changing diapers, doing more feedings, and finding snacks for myself. As my husband's leave from work came to an end, I found myself feeling worried about how I'd get myself and that tiny baby all packed up and out the door for appointments and all the other things we needed to do without having his help. We mostly managed, but that's when my husband started doing the family grocery shopping on his way home from work. It just felt like too much for one person to bring the baby *out* and all the groceries *in*.

My husband, bless his heart, never complained, not even once, about taking up most of the housework in addition to his nine-to-five job, his night shift with the baby, and taking care of both of us whenever he was home. Everything I'd read about postpartum advocated for resting as much as possible, so it didn't even occur to me that my exhaustion, my overwhelm by simple tasks, and my body aches weren't normal. I wasn't depressed; I was happy and enjoying the (tired) bliss of new parenthood, or so I thought. That is, until our pastor's wife knocked on our door with smoked brisket and a tray of macaroni and cheese as part of our church's meal train. Like so many other women in our community, she was graciously bringing us dinner—because new parenthood is a lot, and taking the burden of a meal off our hands would be a blessing. It certainly was a blessing, but the difference between her gift and all the others was what she brought with the meal: a bucket seat with her newborn, Levi, who'd arrived just two-and-a-half weeks earlier than our own son. *And she'd had a C-section!* Yet there she was, standing in our doorway with a fresh meal and pep in her step, whereas I could hardly bring myself to get off the couch.

I brought it up to my husband, who was quick to validate my tiredness—he was tired too—and he pointed out that Levi was older, so a lot would change as our baby grew. *But was two-and-a-half weeks that much of a difference?* After several rounds of "You're not lazy!" and "You're doing great!" and "You're an incredible mom!" I put it out of my mind and carried on, at least as best as I could. Unbeknownst to me, however, I was the only one who had put it out of mind.

At six weeks postpartum, we met our extended family at a pumpkin patch. After walking around for just a few minutes, I felt breathless and faint. I needed to sit down. My back was sore from babywearing, and I was starting to feel like I was getting sick. So, we went home, and I took a three-hour nap.

I thought my behavior was the appropriate response to feeling unwell, but I didn't realize how much of a pattern it had become. My friends started teasing me, shushing each other for "talking too loudly," as I often seemed like I couldn't tolerate commotion and chaos around me and would become snippy and irritable. I just rolled my eyes at them. *They'll understand when they become parents*, I thought. But my best friend, who was already a parent of three, disagreed. She approached me one day and said, "I feel bad for my kids. You won't play with them, and you want them to sit quietly on the couch when we come over. You know that's not realistic, right?"

"I'm just tired, you know how it was," I replied.

"No, I don't, because I don't think it was like that for me. I wonder if you need to see a doctor," she noted, concern in her voice.

"I did. They said everything was great at my six-week appointment."

"And what, exactly, did they say was great?" She raised an eyebrow at me.

"I don't know . . . everything! All the things they checked!"

Her other eyebrow joined the first. "Well, then you need to get checked again," she said, this time with finality in her voice.

It was true there wasn't a whole lot of "checking" going on at my six-week postpartum follow-up visit. They took my blood pressure, handed me a paper depression screening, confirmed that my lochia had stopped, said I wasn't yet due for my Pap, and told me I could return to sex and exercise. That was it, and I was sent on my way. But now it had been six *months* since my son was born and not a lot had changed. I was still following the "rest and relax" advice I'd received in pregnancy, keeping my schedule as light as possible. I only did one thing a day, though sometimes that one thing was simply getting out of bed to make myself a smoothie. Somehow, the task of pulling out the blender, using it, washing it, and then putting it away was enough to completely wipe me out for the rest of the morning. The days of pumpkin patch–type activities were few and far between. *Thank God I have a desk job*, I thought, *because I don't think I could go back to work if I didn't.*

Work, right.

That was when it hit me. *Persistent fatigue? Constipation? Hair loss? Mood swings? Weight changes?* My hand reflexively moved to the space just above my collar bone, toward the bottom of my neck, to check my thyroid. *Swollen thyroid gland?* I scrutinized myself in the mirror, and there it was, unavoidable: a boggy bulge protruding from the base of my neck. My jaw dropped. *How had I missed the signs? How long had this been going on?*

The problem with working in medicine is that I'd become so focused on taking care of other people that I took my own health for granted. It was almost like I knew too much and had seen too much to think that a health crisis would hit me personally. I'd had an uncomplicated pregnancy, an easy delivery, and a healthy baby. But there it was, staring back at me from the mirror. There's an old joke that doctors can heal other people but not themselves, and so it was for me, too, even if only for my stubbornness. I finally made an appointment with my primary care doctor, not because I heeded the advice of all the people around me who could clearly see that something was amiss with my health, but because I finally had accepted it for myself. *Go figure.*

And yet, when I explained the fatigue to my doctor, she was just as reluctant as I was.

"Well, you have small children at home," she said. "Of course you're tired. Parenting is exhausting."

I stared back at her for a moment, taken aback. Admittedly, I wasn't very motivated to have an argument, as it was early, I was tired (as I had just explained), and I was completely naked apart from the gown draped over my shoulders.

"Believe me, this is different," I mumbled. "It's a different kind of tired. And it's been like this for almost a year."

But she didn't believe me, and instead she sent me away with a prescription for a nasal spray, because while I was there, she'd assessed that my nasal passages looked red. *Go figure.*

Stubborn though I was, I had finally accepted for myself that I was struggling with an inflamed thyroid and was newly committed to getting to the bottom of it. So, I found a new doctor with better reviews and booked an appointment with him instead. Fortunately, I got an appointment quickly, and he was much more receptive to my concerns. He ordered a complete thyroid panel and examined my thyroid in the office, agreeing with my assessment that it was swollen and boggy—two signs of inflammation. The final diagnosis, given once my lab results returned a few days later, was postpartum thyroiditis, a very different condition from the tiredness that simply comes with parenting an infant. *Go figure.*

Admittedly, I can't blame the first provider I saw that much because I, too, was hesitant to accept that my experience wasn't normal. Sure, I was a doctor myself with years of experience working with pregnant and postpartum women, but I'd never actually been a mother before. I knew what textbooks said about symptoms, but I'd never personally experienced them. I didn't really know how tired I was supposed to be from waking up every few hours at night because I'd never done it. At what point do you know that it's not just "normal" tired? How old does your baby need to be before "postpartum" stops serving as the explanation for every little symptom?

Fortunately, after a few months of treatment, my thyroid function slowly came back online and my energy along with it. Granted, I was still tired, but it was a different kind of tired. It was the kind of tiredness that comes from keeping up with a crawling baby and lugging a diaper bag and car seat around everywhere you go, not the bone-aching, can't-get-off-the-couch kind of tired. But as I moved farther away from that frustrating medical experience, I started to see my own patients in a new light, particularly the ones who'd previously been to see other providers before seeking out functional medicine care. The ones who'd told me that their doctors proudly announced that their labs were fine, so they were fine. And, of course, the ones whose symptoms started in the weeks, months, and years following pregnancy and childbirth and who, like me, were told it was just a normal part of the postpartum experience. Except that it wasn't, and isn't.

It wasn't and isn't "normal" postpartum, because when I run labs for these patients who, like me, experience unparalleled exhaustion, weight fluctuations, hair loss, and mood changes for months following delivery, I find them to be suffering from thyroid disorders, autoimmune diseases, insulin resistance, hormonal imbalances, and so much more. Sure, they may have small children at home, but they've come to realize that what they are experiencing isn't normal, and it certainly isn't normal *for them*.

As a functional medicine doctor, the majority of my practice is made up of women, particularly in their thirties and forties and typically a few months or years postpartum, dealing with the precise conditions I just listed. I enjoy working with this demographic because I myself fall into it, but I don't send out screeners to prospective patients to ensure they fit into these categories. Rather, women in that season of life seek out functional medicine as an alternative to the traditional model because that model so often fails to diagnose the root cause of symptoms and often also neglects to take these women seriously in the first place. Apart from being considered medical malpractice, negligent care such as this harms both women and their families and is a tremendous problem that needs to be fixed.

Sometimes I'm shocked that so many postpartum women fall through the cracks. After all, it's well-documented in medical research that the hormonal, metabolic, and immunological shifts that occur during pregnancy and postpartum are known triggers for the development of hormonal, metabolic, and immunological disorders. The months and years following childbirth are a high-risk time for new onset of these types of conditions, and this fact is a standard piece of medical education regardless of specialization. Yet, somehow, the medical standard for women is a single follow-up appointment conducted a full six weeks after delivery, with no standard screening labs. If a provider does order blood work, which typically only happens when women experience complications during pregnancy and delivery, it's usually limited to some basic screenings called complete blood count panels (CBC) and comprehensive metabolic panels (CMP). This combination of tests is less detailed than even the annual screening protocols required by some employers, which are covered by most insurance plans.

As a woman and a mother, I believe that the female body is wise and strong and knows how to grow and birth babies. I am fundamentally against the unnecessary overmedicalization of birth. But as a healthcare provider who works with so many sick moms, I also recognize that women are not immune to the development of disease. We live in a broken world, and our bodies are susceptible to illness. At the very least, it is our right to be provided with appropriate postpartum support from medical providers, to be offered the option of laboratory screenings for conditions that are known to be triggered by pregnancy and childbirth, and to be taken seriously when we experience concerning symptoms. Or rather, it should be our right.

There's no such thing as New Mom Syndrome, despite the way healthcare providers sometimes make it seem. Becoming a new mom isn't a disease, and it shouldn't come with debilitating symptoms. Yes, pregnancy and postpartum are physically taxing times, but there's a difference between resting to recover and resting because we *can't* recover, because the real root cause hasn't been found. So, if you have dealt with these same problems, whether they be a missed or delayed diagnosis of a condition that came on after your beautiful baby joined your family; if your doctor neglected to take your symptoms seriously; or if you believe that postpartum and parenting are *just this hard* and you simply need to keep muddling through it all, this book is for you.

Please bear in mind that I don't mean to discount the fact that becoming a new parent, even while in perfect health, can be really, really hard. From the sleeplessness to the unknowns, from feeding schedules to setting one's own needs aside for the sake of another's, it is perfectly acceptable and valid to feel tired and overwhelmed, to experience a wide range of rapidly changing emotions, and to need time getting used to a postpartum body. But what I want to bring to light with this book is that women are smart, and our bodies know when something isn't quite right. When we bring our symptoms to our doctors and they don't believe us, it's not okay. It's not okay for health concerns to be discounted as normal simply because of our season of life. In fact, it's not okay for any symptoms to be considered normal without an appropriate and thorough workup, especially at such a vulnerable and pivotal time as the postpartum period.

In the coming pages I will equip you with the tools you need to understand your postpartum body. We will take a broader look at our medical system and consider how the current setup allows women in a vulnerable position to slip through the cracks. Next, we will take a deeper look at the notorious symptoms of postpartum, ranging from weight changes and hair loss to irregular bleeding and fatigue, outlining what is and is not normal about these experiences.

Considering the possibility of a serious health condition in the delicate time of postpartum can be stressful. However, my goal is not for you to be fearful of what you read in these pages but instead to be empowered. I want you to get the very best possible care so that you can feel your best and enjoy your family without the worry—or reality—of a health crisis.

About Me

If you're going to be taking my advice, I feel it's important for you to know the woman behind the pages. I'm Alexandra MacKillop, a functional medicine doctor with, as you probably have already picked up on, a fiery passion for women's health. I see patients online via telehealth throughout Illinois and a few other Midwestern states, and I write a blog where I share articles about the same sorts of topics you'll find in this book. Prior to entering the world of functional medicine, I ran a nutrition practice where I helped women break up with dieting and learn how to eat their favorite foods without feeling guilty. You'll therefore also find themes about gentle nutrition and making peace with your natural body size in this book.

I earned my bachelor's degree in food science at Purdue University in West Lafayette, where I then completed graduate coursework in clinical nutrition and public health. When I returned to Chicago, I did so in pursuit of my doctoral degree in chiropractic medicine at National University of Health Sciences, where I also completed advanced training in functional medicine with an emphasis on endocrine disorders and fertility. I am also a wife, a mother, a sister, and a cheerleader for all women who want to take their health back into their own hands so they can make decisions for themselves about how they want to care for their bodies. If that describes you, let's get started!

CHAPTER 2

Postpartum Is Forever

Have you ever heard the phrase "the fourth trimester"? The medical community divides the fortyish weeks of pregnancy into three distinct trimesters of twelve or so weeks, which are used to track physical development and milestones of a mother and her baby. For many of us, the tumultuous first trimester in which the baby undergoes the most rapid and dramatic developments brings feelings of sickness and tiredness. Then, in the second trimester, the fog lifts. This period is known for the "glow and show," in which morning sickness often fades, the risk of miscarriage drops between weeks fourteen and twenty-eight, and moms typically can no longer hide their growing joy if they haven't yet shared news of their pregnancy. In the third trimester, notorious for its aches and pains, mom and baby both tend to take on the greatest physical growth. Then—hopefully after reaching full term—the mother delivers her baby, and the three trimesters of pregnancy, with all their glory, finally end.

But as we know, childbirth doesn't magically transform mothers back to their prepregnancy state. Regaining strength and vitality takes time, and we need that time for healing, not just mentally and physically but also socially and emotionally. In a well-intentioned effort to bring awareness to the unique health considerations of the early postpartum period, many have come to refer to the first few months after delivery as "the fourth trimester": another three-month period which is, like the other three, characterized by remarkable physical, emotional, and spiritual changes for new moms. For this reason, we advocate for rest, nourishing food, boundaries, and alleviation of other responsibilities. In other words, the fourth trimester should consist of a time of healing and bonding for the mother and baby as they settle into their new family dynamic and recover from the labor of not just delivery but pregnancy as well. As both a healthcare provider and a mother, I like the idea of referring to these few months as another trimester, considering the profound significance they carry for a woman's health. Creating a term to demarcate this time honors its importance and gravity.

My one criticism of this phrase, however, is that it gives the impression that the postpartum period lasts just a few months. Indeed, some people view postpartum even more narrowly, boiling it down to just a few weeks. As it currently stands, the standard of care in the United States allows up to six weeks of maternity leave for mothers to recover after delivering a baby (or babies) vaginally and up to eight weeks for a C-section delivery. It's after this time frame that healthcare providers invite moms back to their offices to give them the "all clear" for their health—granting them "permission" to return to work, to sex, to exercise, and to leave that whole pregnancy thing in the past. (I personally needed my own doctor to sign a form indicating that I was "fit" to return to work after delivering each of my children.) According to medical coding practices, the diagnosis of "Encounter for routine postpartum follow-up" is no longer used after the point of this six- or eight-week check-in. In medical documentation, after six weeks, it's as though you've never even had a baby!

But these figures factor in just a few small parameters of health, such as whether your uterus returned to its prepregnancy size and whether you're experiencing any bleeding. They do not take into account other important factors, like hormonal shifts or immune system function. Really, they're based more on economics than health: Six and eight weeks are the time frames after which short-term disability providers stop paying for maternity leave, if it was ever a benefit provided at all. But there's nothing magical or special about that six-week time frame. It's an arbitrarily chosen parameter from the healthcare system to ensure that their work has been finished—prescribing birth control, completing an overdue Pap, screening for depression, signing off on the return-to-work form. As I hope to make clear in this chapter, the duration typically used to describe the postpartum period, whether that be six weeks, eight weeks, or twelve weeks, is not based on the realities of postpartum health—because the changes that occur to a woman's body through the process of pregnancy and childbirth have implications for the rest of her life. Postpartum isn't just another trimester, it's forever, and there are real risks to women's health when we don't take that fact into account.

Pregnancy and Your Body in a Nutshell

To understand why pregnancy brings such dramatic health shifts postpartum, and for the rest of our lives, we first need a firm understanding of what all happens during pregnancy itself on a biological level. We obviously didn't need to know this information in order to conceive and carry a healthy baby, considering that our bodies know how to do this perfectly well without any outside help (most of the time). But I believe it's information that moms need to understand so they can cultivate a better attunement to their own bodies for their own well-being and advocate for themselves in a healthcare setting for the rest of their lives. If you've ever been pregnant, you know that your heart is forever changed by that experience. But did you know that your literal heart—and nearly all other aspects of your cardiovascular system—changes during pregnancy too? Blood volume increases by 50 percent throughout a normal pregnancy, and the heart muscle itself along with it.[1] No wonder we feel tired, develop varicose veins, and fall short of breath!

But here's something else that might surprise you: Thyroid function also increases by about 50 percent during pregnancy to keep up with the increased metabolic demands of all that extra blood, all those extra hormones, and, you know, that whole extra person.[2] And thyroid hormones amount to just a drop in the bucket in the context of the major jumps in sex hormones, like estrogen and progesterone, which drive fetal and maternal growth. There's also human chorionic gonadotropin (hCG) itself, the notorious pregnancy hormone that turns the line on pregnancy tests wonderfully pink and leaves many poor moms feeling so sick in the early weeks (or all weeks) of pregnancy.[3] Our brains also change throughout the course of gestation. Is it "mom brain," or is it the dramatic shift in serotonin signaling wrought by pregnancy?[4] Or perhaps the fact that fetal cells don't remain confined to the uterus but migrate all the way to the mother's central nervous system as well, taking up permanent residence in her brain?[5] The moral of the story is that there's a lot more going on through the processes of pregnancy and childbirth than is covered in a typical "birds and bees" conversation. This chapter covers everything else you need to know.

Sex Hormones

Let's begin with sex hormones. Women's reproductive hormones come in two main flavors: estrogen and progesterone. These are the main pregnancy hormones but also the primary hormones that influence a normal menstrual cycle and all the other rhythmic changes that take place throughout a woman's life. In addition to the obvious part about growing a baby, the main difference between a period and a pregnancy is that the body produces these hormones at much higher levels and in different proportions during pregnancy than it does throughout a normal menstrual cycle. As a result, we see changes in the thickness of the uterine lining, in breast development, in body fat proportion, in appetite, and in so many of the other bodily shifts that occur throughout gestation. It's all mediated, at least in part, by these two hormones.

But how does the body know when to make pregnancy levels of estrogen and progesterone versus normal levels? When it comes to overseeing this transition of sex hormones, we can thank the baby. A hormone produced by the fetus—that's hCG—communicates with both the brain and the ovaries to override the normal menstrual cycle signaling and transition to a heightened state of hormone production to sustain the pregnancy. As time goes on and the placenta forms, hCG then begins communicating with this new organ to facilitate hormone production. By the start of the second trimester, the role of the ovaries fades into the background as the placenta pumps out estrogen and progesterone, in addition to all its other essential functions. But with childbirth and delivery, placental production of hormones transitions from nearly 100 percent to 0 percent within moments. Given that the ovaries don't magically come back online when the placenta detaches from the uterine wall, many women experience dramatic symptoms on account of this sudden plummeting of hormones—things like night sweats, fatigue, and mood changes.

During pregnancy, the shifts in estrogen, progesterone, and hCG also coordinate countless other functions of the body beyond just the reproductive organs. These include everything from immune function and thyroid function, metabolism, and even the physical structure of our bodies. So, when sex hormones drop off at delivery, the other bodily systems shift too. Or at least they're supposed to. Let's take a closer look.

Immune System

Beyond the most notable sex hormones, mothers also experience immunological shifts to allow for a healthy baby to grow. Normally, our bodies reject any cells that don't belong to us—think bacteria, yeast, or any other nonhuman cells.

This is a great protective strategy when we're trying to avoid strep throat or ringworm but isn't helpful when we're trying to grow an entirely new human inside our wombs. Out of necessity, the immune system shuts down certain activities to allow the baby to grow. However, there's no free lunch; this immunosuppression also puts pregnant mothers at increased risk of infection. It also may cause problems postpartum by failing to return to its original status or perhaps by rebounding and becoming too aggressive after childbirth, as in the case of autoimmune disease.

The immune system also regulates inflammatory responses in our bodies. Normally, we view inflammation as a bad thing for our health, but during pregnancy we need a certain level of extra inflammation to help coordinate the growth of the baby. But as with the shifts in sex hormones, these elevated inflammation levels may abnormally persist in the postpartum period, making us feel sick (think body aches, swelling, fatigue), or trigger new health problems, like autoimmune diseases, as a result. Persistently elevated levels of inflammation often mimic "normal" postpartum symptoms that we might tend to misattribute to such things as sleeplessness, for example. This becomes another common reason that a doctor might dismiss a new mom's symptoms. Moreover, testing for inflammation levels is not a routine part of pregnancy or postpartum care or even other seasons of life outside the realm of functional medicine. For this reason, doctors in traditional medical settings have a hard time spotting postpartum inflammatory conditions. For moms, knowing about these disorders helps them identify health conditions in themselves where their doctors might otherwise overlook them.

Thyroid Shifts Postpartum

Mediated through the surges of estrogen and progesterone, pregnancy also triggers an uptick in thyroid activity. Because growing a baby takes a lot of resources, the thyroid gland—responsible for coordinating heat production, blood flow, energy use, and new tissue growth—increases its production of thyroid hormones during pregnancy. As a result, the body shifts into what we would normally consider a slightly overactive state throughout the gestational period. In nonpregnant circumstances, this would lead to a diagnosis of hyperthyroidism, though it's necessary and good during pregnancy because of the increased metabolic demands. However, for those with preexisting thyroid disease, whether known and medically managed or still undiagnosed, these pregnancy-mediated changes in thyroid hormone production may lead to complications for pregnant and postpartum mothers. It also may become problematic if all these thyroid shifts don't return to baseline after childbirth, or if they drop back down too far and result in hypothyroidism (an underactive thyroid state), as they often do. Unsurprisingly, pregnancy and childbirth notoriously trigger a new onset of thyroid disease.

The other endocrine shifts occurring postpartum, such as those brought on by breastfeeding, add additional layers of complexity. That's because we also need to consider the problems of inflammation; the nutritional demands of pregnancy and breastfeeding; the physical, mental, and emotional stress of sleeplessness and parenthood; and the toll that these things take on not just thyroid function but also our bodies as a whole. Given this, it's easy to see how things can go awry. Furthermore, considering that the symptoms of thyroid disease so significantly mirror seemingly "normal" postpartum experiences, we clearly see how misdiagnosis—and missed diagnosis—can happen too.

Metabolic Shifts Postpartum

Remember that conversation we had earlier about progesterone and metabolism? There's much more to that story. Your prenatal provider probably talked with you at some point about weight gain. To the chagrin of many postpartum women struggling to lose their baby weight, we do need to gain weight during pregnancy. This makes sense considering what is required to sustain a burgeoning new life, to carry the weight of that second person, and to accumulate resources for future breastfeeding. But have you ever wondered what goes on behind the scenes to increase these tissue stores? Perhaps you can relate to my experience in pregnancy, in which I gained over fifteen pounds in the first trimester despite changing nothing at all about my eating or exercise habits. If anything, my appetite had decreased from nausea—so I was surprised by how quickly my weight changed considering that my eating habits hadn't.

Insulin, a hormone designed to keep blood sugar levels under control, largely drives these weight changes in pregnancy. As it turns out, the rules about insulin completely change during pregnancy to promote the process of taking the calories we were already eating and storing them up as body fat for later. This usually resolves postpartum, following the delivery of the placenta, but not always. As a result, postpartum problems like insulin resistance, metabolic syndrome, and even type 2 diabetes can develop in women who were otherwise healthy prior to pregnancy. It's also important to note that while a mother's health status before conception certainly influences the risk of developing metabolic dysfunction postpartum, the weight shifts that occur while pregnant largely result from pregnancy-induced hormone recalibration as opposed to maternal eating and exercise behavior. Remember that during pregnancy the baby puts on weight quickly by design, which means that the mother's own metabolism also needs to change to help them grow and remain healthy. As a result, the mother herself also experiences changes in how her body processes food—especially sugars—during pregnancy. While this phenomenon should resolve postpartum, it doesn't always.

The shifts in our bodies' stress-regulation systems that occur during pregnancy and postpartum also complicate the metabolic puzzle. Cortisol, the main stress hormone, plays a role not just in regulating stress but also in coordinating sleep (which we know looks very different with a newborn than without one), metabolism, energy levels, and body weight. Our bodies prefer a very tightly controlled pattern of cortisol production, but during pregnancy, levels increase sometimes up to triple the normal amount.[6] Like the other metabolic events, this increase is necessary and good during pregnancy but causes problems when levels don't return exactly to baseline after birth. If elevated, high cortisol brings the same side effects to the life of a postpartum mom that it would bring during pregnancy—symptoms like swelling, blood sugar changes, mood swings, fatigue, weight gain, and so on.

Structural Shifts Postpartum

Next, there's the obvious physical piece. As a pregnant mama's belly expands, her organs rearrange to make room for a growing baby by relaxing and stretching the abdominal muscles. To provide for such dramatic expansion, the gluteal muscles also must deactivate. Along with changes to sex hormones, immune function, and metabolism, pregnancy brings a complete restructuring of a mother's musculoskeletal system. Hormones take part of the credit for this phenomenon too. In the case of physical structure, a hormone called relaxin—appropriately named—relaxes ligaments, allowing the bones of the pelvis to shift and rearrange, widening to accommodate a changing gait and to eventually allow passage of the baby during vaginal delivery. Progesterone plays a role here, too, relaxing and lengthening muscles, including those that hold tension in veins (causing varicose veins to develop), maintain sphincters (like the esophageal sphincter, the relaxation of which often leads to heartburn), and make up the gastrointestinal tract (slowing down gut motility and potentially leading to constipation, hemorrhoids, and more).

While the repositioning of all our bodily structures is good and arguably essential for the progression of a healthy pregnancy, it also creates some complications. After all, the hip bones connect to the leg bones and the leg bones connect to the knee bones, possibly creating problems with gait patterns that can lead to pain and injury. Stretchy joints certainly can go too far! But the relaxin-related risk of overextending joints isn't the only reason for injury. Stretching and loss of strength in the muscles that normally hold the pelvis in place create instability that can lead to sprains, strains, and pain. Even though most obstetric providers recommend a period of rest following delivery, they miss an important point: Rested muscles lose strength, and that strength doesn't magically return simply because six weeks have passed. Mamas need, and deserve, tailored pelvic rehab to support their recovery. But that's a conversation for chapter 10.

Bringing It Back Home

When it comes to hormone regulation, metabolic control, immune system function, and structural changes, there's nothing quite like pregnancy. Realistically, if the changes that occur during pregnancy were to take place in a nonpregnant woman, most doctors would have no difficulty seeing the problem. But in pregnancy, we say it's all well and good! And it certainly is a good, necessary, amazing design. The systems of the body were made to produce all these biochemical shifts and then reverse them one by one as the baby and placenta leave a mother's body. However, these necessary reversals don't always take place after birth, and we then see issues like metabolic dysfunction and autoimmune disease. In other cases, the gun loaded by genetics has its trigger pulled by the intense experiences of pregnancy and childbirth, akin to flipping a switch that creates a new problem that never should have occurred in the first place. This is true no matter how long the pregnancy lasted—whether to full term or ending unfortunately in miscarriage.

Our bodies are smart, but so are we. We know when something is amiss with our health, and even though childbirth will always both transform us and tire us out, there comes a point when pregnancy-related changes stop being normal and instead become problematic. We ultimately end up helping ourselves when we know what to expect and how to differentiate when our experiences are not to be expected. Whether it's a matter of bringing our symptoms to our doctors' attention so they can better help us or simply asking for a higher degree of screening and care postpartum, knowing how our bodies work is an ally and an asset for caring well for ourselves throughout pregnancy and into motherhood.

CHAPTER 3

How and Why Healthcare Providers Get It Wrong

In 2023, physicians at Dayton's Wright State University published a case study about a twenty-four-year-old woman—let's call her Rachel—who, like me, received a diagnosis of postpartum thyroiditis. Sadly, Rachel's case differs from mine in that she delivered but then ultimately lost her baby following an emergency cesarean performed at twenty-four weeks gestation. Following the sudden delivery, Rachel developed numerous symptoms classically associated with thyroid disorders, including weakness, fatigue, cold intolerance, hair loss, insomnia, and mood shifts. However, because her pregnancy ended in miscarriage rather than with a living infant, numerous doctors overlooked the relationship between her symptoms and the risks brought on by her recent pregnancy. Before receiving a referral for a rheumatologist and finally an endocrinologist (aka hormone specialist) who published a narrative of her condition, Rachel was first referred for psychiatric testing under the assumption that her symptoms resulted from a mood disorder.[1]

It's not that doctors necessarily believed that her symptoms were "all in her head," or at least that's what I am choosing to believe (the publication was unclear about the initial assessment). Rather, I'm assuming that the misdiagnosis of Rachel's postpartum thyroiditis came for the same reasons that mine did: an unfortunate combination of provider error, personal misgivings, and cultural factors. When considering the problem of healthcare providers dismissing postpartum symptoms as normal despite their debilitating nature, one of the most important questions to ask is how and why this happens. After all, the postpartum thyroiditis that affected Rachel and me is certainly not the only health condition triggered by pregnancy and childbirth, nor is it the most common. As I'll explain in this chapter, the gap in diagnosis and treatment of postpartum health concerns stems from provider error, yes, but it also depends on cultural, political, and social factors as well as behaviors of the women themselves. Answering this question of why leads us directly into the solution for preventing it from happening to you and your loved ones, or from happening *again*.

Why Doctors Dismiss Symptoms as "Normal"

Even if you haven't experienced a misdiagnosis yourself, you've probably heard of it happening to someone you know. That's because diagnostic error is a huge problem in our medical system. As defined in *Science*, the journal of the American Association for the Advancement of Science, diagnostic errors are "inaccurate assessments of a patient's root cause of illness," and an estimated "800,000 Americans die or are permanently disabled by diagnostic errors each year."[2] This amounts to roughly 5 percent of adults experiencing misdiagnosis annually, and authors note that most people will experience this phenomenon at least once in their lifetime. With postpartum specifically, diagnostic errors can reach as high as 33 percent, as stated in a 2024 review article published in the *Journal of Clinical Medicine*.[3]

But why all the confusion? If postpartum health conditions are so well-documented in the research (which they are—more on that later), how do they get missed so often? From a provider standpoint, these errors come down to lack of clear role differentiation among care providers, deficiencies in medical training, the need for better standardization of postpartum follow-up protocols, provider bias, and time constraints wrought by a shortage of healthcare providers.

One reason for misdiagnosis comes from the lack of clarity in whose role it is to screen for such problems. In hospital settings, obstetricians typically only follow up with patients once—the day after an otherwise uncomplicated delivery. The mother is then discharged from the hospital and isn't invited back to her provider's office for a full six weeks. In some cases, the gynecological follow-up doesn't occur for an entire year, with the postpartum checkup provided instead by a primary care doctor who may or may not have ever examined the patient while she was pregnant. As we will get to in a moment, training in postpartum care leaves much to be desired among perinatal specialists and even more so among primary care doctors. A 2021 research study regarding the experiences of primary care physicians managing postpartum care found that the ability of these providers to diagnose, treat, and properly care for postpartum mothers was influenced by everything from prior training to personal childcare experience and access to resource materials in their practice. At the same time, they were also limited by "inadequate handover of care from the specialists," meaning that in many cases the primary care doctors never had the opportunity to collaborate with the attending obstetric providers before following up with their patients.[4] Lack of communication creates problems in all marriages but especially so in the high-stakes union of medical specialists for the purpose of patient case management.

Recognizing the problem with this lack of care continuity, Weill Cornell Medicine and NewYork-Presbyterian Hospital received funding for a 2023 project designed to improve postpartum health outcomes through a six-month program of doula-delivered postpartum support, helping patients with everything from blood pressure management to nutrition and mental health.[5] While doulas most certainly play an important role in supporting mothers during pregnancy, delivery, and the postpartum period, they lack the required scope of practice to test for and treat postpartum health conditions. At the end of the day, a doctor must be the one to make an accurate diagnosis. But like the specialized, support-focused training of doulas, highly trained physicians often spend most of their time preparing for their own highly specialized roles, like performing surgeries. This comes at the expense of everyday health education for mothers with uncomplicated deliveries.

The medical training of obstetric providers unfortunately also often minimizes the complexity of uncomplicated deliveries, failing to recognize that a mother who safely delivered a baby may still experience a health crisis related to her pregnancy. I once attended a birth in which the obstetrician's postpartum instructions to the birthing mother came in the form of six short parting words: "No douching, no sex, no tampons." In this patient's case, that sentence was her final encounter with that provider for the rest of her life, as he retired shortly after attending her baby's birth. Most medical providers don't provide much more than that, if they provide that much at all, nor are they encouraged throughout the course of their training to routinely counsel patients regarding these important postpartum issues. The 2022 NIH publication "Postpartum Care of the New Mother" outlines just four "common" postpartum concerns: postpartum blues, intimate partner violence, incontinence, and hemorrhoids.[6] Plainly missing from the list are thyroid disorders (affecting up to 10 percent of women);[7] autoimmune diseases, which are 11 percent higher among women who have had children compared to those who haven't;[8] as well as adrenal, metabolic, and nutritional disorders. Likewise, despite the well-known relationship between childbirth and disorders of the pelvic floor, research studies have shown that "prenatal counseling of pelvic floor dysfunction risk is lacking at all levels of obstetrical training."[9] Additionally, many obstetric providers do not even receive training in perinatal depression screening,[10] despite this being one of the top reasons for the postpartum visit in the first place.[11] Ultimately, doctors aren't going to diagnose what they don't test for, and they aren't going to test for disorders they were never trained to screen.

Awareness of these postpartum health concerns, both in the medical community as well as outside of it, has grown in recent decades. However, medical practices are driven by policy, and there's a marked lack of standardization in postpartum follow-up protocols. I experienced this myself after the birth of my first child versus my second. The first time around, my midwife called me two weeks after delivery to screen for depression, and I was offered a paper questionnaire at my six-week follow-up visit. The second time, delivering with a different medical group, I didn't receive a screening at all, except from my daughter's pediatrician, with an outside charge of twenty-five dollars for the service. Realistically, knowing that the screening wasn't covered by insurance, many women would understandably decline to complete the form altogether.

This isn't to say that there is a lack of effort to drive change. Take the screening in the pediatrician's office, for example: This provider was my child's, not my own, but knowing the risks and the prevalence of perinatal depression, she offered to screen *me* anyway. However, by today's standards, it's too little, too late. The World Health Organization (WHO) recommended a minimum of *four* postpartum visits to all new mothers within the first six weeks back in 2013, and in 2018, the American College of Obstetricians and Gynecologists (ACOG) recommended a twelve-week program of comprehensive care beginning no later than three weeks postpartum. But alas, as of 2026, the standard for US mothers is still a single visit a month and a half after delivery, and this visit includes a whopping *zero* laboratory screenings as a standard of care. Moreover, due to physician productivity pressures and time constraints, obstetricians normally don't have time for such extensive examinations even if we were to successfully raise the bar; after all, the average length of a primary care visit in the US, as reported in 2021, was a breezy eighteen minutes.[12]

Why Moms Dismiss Their Own Symptoms

It's undeniable that provider error in patient diagnosis is a big problem, though because of inertia in care standards and the context in which most physicians are working, we can't blame the doctors entirely. They need support to be able to do their jobs well. At the same time, no doctor can help a patient who fails to recognize in themselves the fact that help is needed. A 2021 ACOG report states that up to 40 percent of women don't even attend their six-week postpartum visit![13] Mamas—no matter how inconvenient it would be, no matter how much you think you're "fine," no matter how much you'd rather get that hour of sleep—please, please, *please* take advantage of the opportunity for someone to help make sure you're as healthy as possible after childbirth. It's so easy to prioritize your beautiful new baby. But your health is not to be taken for granted. Even if your experience seems to match the struggle of commiserating mom friends, even if postpartum complications seem rare in your circles, go get checked out! Your baby needs you to be healthy too.

The Role of Culture, Politics, and Legislation in Postpartum Healthcare

One of the most important shifts I've witnessed in recent years is a growing awareness of—and, finally, open conversation about—just how hard motherhood truly is. As more women faced pressure to return to work in the '80s and '90s, it brought with it a cultural narrative of "bouncing back," setting arbitrary standards for how long it was considered acceptable to rest, recover, and adjust to such a tremendous lifestyle change.

The timeline set, however, was far too short. Even in uncomplicated births, the physical demands of childbirth, layered with the invisible labor of household management and the intense emotional, cognitive, and physical strain of returning to work, often without support, created an unsustainable burden. Thankfully, we're naming this reality now. But I've seen a strange paradox emerge among my patients and online: In recognizing the challenges of postpartum, we've begun to normalize the struggle itself. Yes, in the US we make postpartum adjustment far harder than we need to, particularly in light of socioeconomic disparities and outright lack of healthcare coverage. But even within that harsh reality, there's a threshold where "hard" becomes too hard. In the past, the cultural message was to buck up or get fired. But now, even our acceptance and acknowledgment have become pathological: *Of course postpartum is hard. Of course you're tired. Of course you aren't sleeping—what new mom does?* But sometimes it's not just a case of being tired simply because you had a baby. Instead, it's Rachel. And it's me. And maybe it's you too.

Reframing Postpartum Health

Despite recommendations for better medical support, we're still dealing with a substandard level of care in the US. But you don't have to fall through the cracks; you can demand (politely, of course) better for yourself. Advocating in a healthcare setting can sound scary. We often see doctors as authority figures, and we fear that they will dismiss us, label us, and perhaps rudely remind us that they "know more than your Google search." Perhaps you were raised to trust and not question doctors or anyone else. Maybe you don't even really believe that your symptoms are all that bad but this book has made you wonder if you should make an appointment just in case. Let me assuage your fears for a moment. Remember that doctors:

1. Want to help you. The vast majority pursued a career in medicine because of the desire to do exactly that.
2. Are people too. Talk to them the way you would in any other conversation among equal parties. See past the white coat and remember that doctors also need to eat, sleep, and receive medical care for their own health problems.
3. Also lack support. Our medical system makes the job of physicians unnecessarily hard in the same way that it undersupports patients. Most doctors are strapped for time, are stressed, and are doing the best they can with the tools they've been given.
4. Are hired by you to provide a service. I don't advocate for going into medical appointments armed and ready for a fight, but remember that *you* are paying *them*. If you don't like the care provided, get a new doctor!

Before you have the chance to listen to any doctors, however, you first need to listen to yourself. Pay attention to what your body is telling you. While you certainly should expect some shifts in your body and sense of well-being in the months and years following childbirth, don't just automatically accept them as your new normal. Pay attention to each system of your body and how your health in that area compares to what you experienced before becoming pregnant. Here's a guide for checking in with yourself to stay on top of your health. I recommend completing this self-checkup on a monthly basis for the first year of your child's life:

- **Integumentary system (hair, skin, nails):** Have I noticed changes to my hair texture or color or to the amount I lose in the shower? Am I experiencing dry or oily skin? Do I have new or changing moles, new skin tags, or skin texture? Do I have new rashes, acne, or sores that won't heal? Are my nails brittle or dry? Do they have changes in texture or color?
- **Musculoskeletal system:** Have I noticed changes in my mobility or walking patterns? Am I experiencing pain? Do I struggle to recover after a workout? Have I developed postural changes? When I stand in front of a mirror, does my body appear symmetrical?
- **Nervous system:** How is my mental health? Am I more down and depressed, or perhaps anxious and irritable, than usual? Do I have the same clarity of thought, memory, and processing ability that I used to? Am I experiencing headaches? Can I hear and see as easily as I used to? How is my dexterity? Can I perceive the texture of objects with my fingertips (and toes) the same way I used to? Do I fall asleep and stay asleep easily? Can I manage daily stress as well as I used to?
- **Endocrine system:** Is my weight unintentionally or unexpectedly changing, or failing to respond to efforts that worked well in the past? Do I have difficulty regulating my body temperature? Do I experience fatigue

or bursts of energy? Am I hungrier or thirstier than usual?

- **Cardiovascular system:** Do my hands and feet feel cold? Do I feel dizzy, such as when I stand up after sitting or lying down? Do I feel pain, pressure, or tightness in my chest? Do I notice any swelling in my body (particularly in my legs)?
- **Lymphatic/immune system:** Am I getting sick more than usual? Do I have a persistent cough, runny nose, or itchy or watery eyes? Does my face appear swollen in the morning? Does my clothing leave indentations in my skin? Do I notice any lumps or bumps in my neck, armpits, or groin?
- **Respiratory system:** Do I feel particularly winded during exercise? Do my lips or nose appear blue? Does my breathing at rest satisfy me? Do I wake up gasping for air?
- **Digestive system:** Do I have daily bowel movements? Have my stools changed in texture, size, color, or frequency? Do I experience bloating, abdominal pain, or cramping surrounding bowel movements? Do I burp or pass gas more than usual? Do I have heartburn, nausea, or vomiting? Is there blood, mucus, or undigested food in my stool?
- **Urinary system:** Am I experiencing urinary urgency or incontinence when coughing, jumping, sneezing, or laughing? Does my urine spray when I void? Do I have the sensation of complete emptying of my bladder? Is it difficult for me to initiate urination? Is there pain or pressure? Is there blood in my urine?

- **Reproductive system:** Do I experience pelvic pain with physical activity, using the bathroom, or sex? Are there changes in sensation to my vulva or vagina, including pressure, protrusion, or prickling sensations? If my periods have returned, are they heavier or lighter, more or less painful, more or less frequent, or more or less regular compared to prepregnancy? Do I notice signs and symptoms of ovulation? Changes in discharge? Changes in libido? Have I performed my monthly breast self-examination? If I am breastfeeding, do I have any concerns about milk supply, quality, or production?

If at any point you identify an abnormality, I recommend making an appointment with your healthcare provider and plainly stating your concerns. Here's an example of how to share your concerns and advocate for care:

- "I had a baby ___ months ago, and since then, I've noticed some changes to my health. They are: ________."
- "I've done some research, and I'm concerned about __________. I would love to know what you think might be causing these symptoms."
- "Because of my concerns, I would like the following tests run in addition to any other diagnostics that you recommend: ______________."

Most healthcare providers will gladly honor these requests and take the initiative themselves to run the appropriate tests when you share your concerns. You don't need to become a physician yourself just to make sure you get quality healthcare. However, I always recommend that women educate themselves as much as they can so they can make sure their symptoms aren't overlooked. Subsequent chapters of this book will provide additional information regarding the types of tests and evaluations that you may want to ask your doctor about, depending on the nature of your symptoms.

Become the Change You Wish to See in Healthcare

As we reviewed earlier, the current standard of a single postpartum visit at six weeks is insufficient to appropriately screen and capture the breadth of potential health concerns women experience after giving birth. I recommend taking the recommendations provided by the WHO and ACOG into account and working with your provider before giving birth to create a postpartum support plan. Bear in mind that not all these visits need to be completed with an obstetric provider or midwife; instead, you can put together a team of healthcare professionals to support you over the course of your first year postpartum. These can include the provider who attends your birth, your primary care doctor, any specialists you have seen, mental health providers, lactation consultants, physical therapists, chiropractors, naturopaths, functional medicine doctors, dietitians, acupuncturists, and more. Here's what I recommend as a starting point:

1. Meet with someone within two weeks of giving birth. This may be a simple check-in with your therapist, a chiropractic adjustment, or a telehealth wellness check with your midwife. Make as many appointments as

feels appropriate to you, but I recommend a minimum of one.

2. Complete your regularly scheduled six-week follow-up with the physician or midwife who attended your birth. In addition to the physical examinations and testing provided, request that your doctor also order routine blood labs (outlined below) as a preventive screening. If your OB/midwife declines to order these tests, make an appointment with your primary care doctor so they can order the tests for you. Request to repeat these labs at six months and one year postpartum as well, as postpartum health conditions such as thyroid disease commonly appear several months after delivery.[14] In addition to lab testing, I also recommend that all women receive a referral for at least ten sessions of pelvic floor physical therapy to rehabilitate pelvic muscles following the physical trauma of pregnancy and childbirth. (In France, the standard of care for all women is twenty visits, but if you need this much, your physical therapist will tell you.)[15] For more on the need for this, see chapter 10, "Pelvic Floor Dysfunction."
3. Complete additional visits with healthcare providers as wellness touchpoints every three months for the first year in addition to the two-week and six-week visits.
4. Meet with all the providers you were seeing prior to delivery (i.e., mental health therapist, chiropractor, or any other medical specialists) at least once in the first twelve weeks postpartum for examination and to establish a treatment plan, if necessary.

Routine Lab Tests to Request Postpartum

The following lab tests are usually included as part of an annual wellness examination. I recommend they all be completed around six weeks postpartum and again by the six- and twelve-month marks:

- Complete blood count (CBC)
- Comprehensive metabolic panel (CMP)
- Hemoglobin A1C
- Fasting insulin
- Thyroid panel, including thyroid-stimulating hormone (TSH), free and total T3, free and total T4, and thyroglobulin (Tg)/thyroid peroxidase (TPO) antibodies
- Morning cortisol
- Iron, ferritin, and total iron binding capacity
- Zinc serum
- Magnesium, red blood cell (RBC)
- Vitamin D
- Vitamin B_{12}/folate
- OmegaCheck (omega-3 and -6 fatty acids)

You might be wondering why cholesterol screening[16] and C-reactive protein (inflammation)[17] are not included on this list. Both of these values normally become elevated during pregnancy and may remain so for several months postpartum. Breastfeeding may produce additional changes to levels of cholesterol and inflammation throughout the duration of lactation, so I don't recommend routinely testing them until at least three months after weaning or until your next regularly scheduled wellness exam.[18]

Understanding why providers so often miss postpartum health conditions highlights the need for self-advocacy in the postpartum period. But when you see your own symptoms clearly, you gain the power to seek care with confidence. In the next chapter, we'll take a deeper look at the most common postpartum symptoms, exploring what's to be expected, what's not, and when to speak up so you can stop second-guessing and finally feel like yourself again.

CHAPTER 4

Let's Play "Normal" or "Not Normal"

In a recent conversation, my friend Jessica shared with me that she experienced a mild case of postpartum depression after her third baby was born. "But," she said, "if you'd asked me at the time whether or not I felt like I was depressed, I would've said no." She explained that she'd previously experienced depression as a university student, and her mental health in parenthood didn't feel anywhere close to that. Rather, becoming a parent felt like finally finding fulfillment in life. On paper, though, things weren't as black-and-white—at least not when she reconsidered them several years down the road.

Jessica shared with me that in her postpartum experience, she was fully functional: She strapped her baby into a carrier and hauled her other kids to the pool, the library, the playground, and everywhere else they needed to go. Her hair wasn't washed, and her clothes didn't match. "But, hey," she said, "we made it out of the house, and that's enough to ask of a postpartum mama, isn't it?"

But as she reflected on that feeling of "to heck with my appearance, who cares what people think?" Jessica wondered if it had lasted a bit too long. Of course, none of the concerns she listed were moral issues but instead hygiene concerns she'd previously kept up with, like getting haircuts or shaving her legs, that took longer than she expected to make it back into her regular routine. "That," she mentioned, "and I didn't go through the trouble of swapping out my maternity clothes with regular clothes until my daughter was over a year old because I simply did not care enough until the leggings literally would not stay up anymore!" It wasn't just the shift in her appearance though. She said she felt emotionally flat, unmotivated. She neglected her previous hobbies not because she didn't have enough time but because she didn't feel creative or interested in them the same way.

Indeed, parenting is tiring for everyone. Sleeplessness affects our moods. On top of that, the self-talk we might use to justify lack of upkeep in appearance is probably true—it's doubtful that anyone *does* notice things like day-three hair. Besides, if you asked Jessica, she would have said she was happy. But although she was happy, Jessica suspected something was off because she just wasn't herself and hadn't been for quite some time. Maybe you can relate.

Jessica told me that a few months after her daughter turned one and stopped nursing, her demeanor shifted. She said, a sparkle now in her eyes, "I suddenly had more drive, more motivation, more pep in my step. The real me had returned, and I hadn't realized she'd gone." She recounted how she felt like she'd woken up from a deep sleep, looked at herself in the mirror one day, and was horrified by the state of her hair. It was like a switch flipped, and she immediately went out to buy a few new shirts and even pulled her old underwire bras out of storage. She started wearing makeup again, simply because she finally felt like it.

Of course, I'm not suggesting that it's right or wrong to wear your hair up in a bun or down, to wear makeup or glasses, to embrace or disregard fashion trends. But there was a distinct difference for Jessica between her interests and motivations in the first year of her daughter's life compared to the second. It's only because of this shift that the thought ever occurred to her that something might have been a little off with her health.

I know for a fact that Jessica is not alone in being unsure about whether a health experience is or was normal. While the symptoms she experienced lifted without leaving too much to show for them, the same isn't true for everyone. For some women, undiagnosed postpartum depression is more than a haircut or lack thereof. It can be, and often is, completely devastating, affecting everything from necessary self-care to relationships, bonding with the infant, and work performance. It's a quality-of-life issue and, in some horrible cases, truly a matter of life and death. Moreover, even when it brings gut-wrenching, debilitating symptoms, it still can come on insidiously, leaving both women and their doctors questioning whether something is or was ever truly wrong.

In this chapter, I want to equip you, dear mama, with a more straightforward understanding of what is and is not normal when it comes to symptoms. I don't want you to sit at home for months with your hair falling out, your stomach tied in knots, your lips chapped and cracked and peeling. I don't want you to fear ridicule or experience a delay in care. Yes, becoming a parent is hard and tiring. Sleeplessness is hard. Recovery from pregnancy and childbirth is hard. But when normal hard becomes something more, don't let yourself—or anyone else—chalk it up to "being postpartum," missing the fact of something else going on under the surface. You deserve better!

What's Normal and What's Not

If you were to google "normal postpartum symptoms," I'd guarantee that you could find a blog somewhere attributing virtually any symptom to the condition of postpartum. In fact, the Cleveland Clinic, a renowned online medical reference, lists everything from pain to exhaustion, constipation to night sweats, and hair loss to weight changes as "normal" postpartum symptoms.[1] As a healthcare provider reading this list, I am tempted to laugh because such symptoms are so vague and lacking in context that it's pretty much impossible to assess whether or not they are normal. Each individual item on the list is just as likely to be pathological as it is to be expected.

Take pain, for example, which makes it onto most postpartum symptom lists. Where is the pain? Is it perineal pain? Breast pain? Abdominal pain? Is it from a vaginal tear? Mastitis? An inflamed gallbladder? (Postpartum women are at increased risk for developing this condition.) Or what about constipation? This could be a side effect of narcotic medications administered via an epidural catheter during delivery, a sign of hypothyroidism, the result of pelvic organ prolapse, a consequence of undereating, or dehydration. There are so many normal causes, and yet so many abnormal causes at the same time. How is a woman to know? How is she to get the care she needs if her doctor just chalks it up to being part of the package of parenthood?

Throughout the remainder of this chapter, we will explore the most common postpartum symptoms and experiences—which often receive the default diagnosis of "normal"—and outline when they truly are and are not. For each, when the symptoms do reflect a normal experience, we will review strategies you can use at home to manage them. At the end of the chapter, you will find questionnaires to help you understand if your own pattern of symptoms points to an underlying health condition that needs investigation. You can use the results of these questionnaires when referencing the subsequent, condition-specific chapters of this book. As far as underlying problems outside of "normal" postpartum that may cause the symptoms, we'll address those in more detail in part 2.

Postpartum Symptoms

Please note that the symptom list in this section is not exhaustive and merely outlines some of the most common, non-emergency experiences in the first year after childbirth. Please always advocate for a thorough workup of your symptoms from your own healthcare providers. When considering the treatment options outlined in this chapter or elsewhere in the book, always discuss with your healthcare provider before starting anything new. Please also keep in mind that this chapter references symptoms that are commonly understood to be normal during the postpartum period, but some symptoms are never normal. If you experience chest pain, trouble breathing, heavy bleeding with clots larger than the size of an egg, extreme pain of any kind, or anything else that worries you, go to the emergency room right away.

Aches and Pains (Body Aches and Joint Pain)

Joint pain may normally occur postpartum as the hormone relaxin, which creates joint laxity during pregnancy, clears from the bloodstream. Joints that reposition during pregnancy and delivery—especially those of the pelvis, hips, and legs—are more likely to become sore postpartum, though this shouldn't last more than a week or two. Red and swollen joints are less likely to be the result of normal processes. Additionally, if the joint pain debilitates you to the point of, say, preventing you from moving around normally or exercising, there's likely a deeper issue that needs to be addressed. In addition to the conditions outlined in part 2 of this book, joint pain may also result from dehydration, low estrogen levels wrought by breastfeeding, or infections.

At-Home Treatment for Normal Aches and Pains (Breastfeeding-Safe)

- **Ibuprofen:** This medication is available over the counter in 200 mg and 400 mg tablets, dosed every four to six hours. It is not recommended to use the maximum dose (2,400 mg) daily for more than a few days, and you should always take it under the guidance of a doctor. If you experience body aches that don't improve with the use of ibuprofen or require ibuprofen to manage after a few days, it is essential that you have a thorough workup from a physician.

What about acetaminophen? Acetaminophen, unlike ibuprofen, may temporarily relieve pain but is not an anti-inflammatory drug. It consequently does not work as well for pain relief that results from "normal" postpartum. It also carries more significant risks to the liver, and it transfers to breastmilk at higher rates than ibuprofen. Acetaminophen is often recommended to use for pain relief for the purpose of spacing out doses of ibuprofen. However, if you need to take enough pain relievers for a long enough period of time that spacing of this nature is required, it's a sign that something more significant is going on, and it is essential that you have a thorough workup from a physician.

- **Magnesium glycinate:** This is one of the most bioavailable forms of magnesium, which works well for aches and pains. In my practice, I recommend patients take 300–400 mg of magnesium with a small snack before bed.
- **Omega-3 fatty acids:** These decrease the production of pain-causing inflammatory chemicals.[2] I typically recommend 4,000–6,000 mg daily to my patients and monitor blood levels to make sure we don't exceed a safe intake.
- **Bromelain:** This enzyme, naturally found in pineapple, breaks down inflammation in body tissues.[3] For the purpose of muscle pain, it should be taken on an empty stomach rather than with food.

Numbness/Tingling and Swelling

If you've ever had your arm fall asleep after a period of unuse, you've experienced that familiar pins-and-needles feeling, also known as paresthesia. This may occur in hands, feet, arms, and legs in the first few days postpartum due to fluid retention. It also may feel like a vague sense of numbness in the fingertips. It should not last longer than a few days, if at all. Swelling, especially asymmetrical swelling, should always be evaluated by a doctor. Many women also notice that their hands, feet, and face appear mildly puffy for a few days postpartum. In addition to the conditions outlined in part 2 of this book, numbness, tingling, and swelling may result from nerve compression, postpartum preeclampsia, blood clots, or infections, all of which may be emergencies.

At-Home Treatment for Numbness/Tingling and Swelling (Breastfeeding-Safe)

- **Lymphatic drainage:** This technique helps move and eliminate the fluid that causes swelling and any associated numbness or tingling. Consider making an appointment for a gentle massage, such as that provided by a lymphatic drainage specialist.
- **Dry brushing:** Similar to lymphatic drainage massage, dry brushing is an at-home technique for moving lymph and reducing swelling. However, the distinction is that it is performed with a soft-bristled brush on bare skin.
- **Saunas:** Saunas promote detoxification and movement of lymph. Their use also helps eliminate biological waste, such as old pregnancy hormones, which promote fluid retention.

Hair Loss

In the medical community, most specialists agree that postpartum hair loss is normal; however, there are numerous differing opinions as to why it occurs. While some hair loss, typically around three months postpartum, is to be expected, persistent, patchy, or profound hair loss is not. Likewise, hair loss that continues past twelve months postpartum should be evaluated.[4] In addition to the conditions outlined in part 2 of this book, hair loss may result from sex hormone imbalances, heavy metal or other toxin exposure, allergic reactions, skin infections, and more.

At-Home Treatment for Normal Hair Loss (Breastfeeding-Safe)

- **Brushing and styling techniques:** Brushes that pull hair strands increase hair loss due to stress on the root. Consider gently detangling hair in the shower using a wide-toothed comb and conditioner. Softly pat wet hair with a towel instead of tousling it. Avoid hot tools.
- **Scalp massage:** Gentle scalp massage increases blood flow to the hair follicles, which need oxygen and nutrients to grow. Eleven to twenty minutes of daily massage supports hair regrowth.[5]
- **Vitamins:** While taking prenatal vitamins is not a magic solution for all types of hair loss, appropriate supplementation helps prevent the development of nutrient deficiencies that may lead to hair loss. I recommend that my patients continue supplementation with prenatal vitamins for at least three months after breastfeeding cessation.

Insomnia

Have you ever heard the advice to sleep when your baby sleeps? That is assuming *you actually can fall asleep*. While sleep deprivation is often considered normal postpartum, if everyone in your house is sleeping at night—and *you* can't—you are likely dealing with insomnia, and this is not normal. In addition to the conditions outlined in part 2 of this book, insomnia may result from sex hormone imbalances or use of some medications or supplements.

At-Home Treatment for Insomnia (Breastfeeding-Safe)

- **Magnesium L-Threonate:** This is the best form of magnesium available to be utilized by the brain for promoting sleep and calming anxiety. Research shows that supplementation with 1,000 mg improves sleep duration and quality as well as daytime functioning.[6]

Fatigue

You should expect some tiredness in the postpartum period due to the physical toll of pregnancy and childbirth. In this context, fatigue refers to not just a feeling of sleepiness but of whole-body tiredness. Fatigue may be described as a sensation of heavy limbs, moving through mud, or like you've had your batteries taken out. Normal fatigue improves with rest and sleep. If you don't feel more energized after a period of R&R, or if the fatigue persists longer than a week or two, it may signal an underlying problem. Check out the targeted strategies related to nutrition, rest, and exercise in chapter 13, "A Healthy Post-partum Plan," to prevent fatigue from getting out of control.

Brain Fog

Brain fog refers to having a hard time thinking clearly. This may manifest as forgetfulness, difficulty understanding abstract concepts, lack of focus, or even the sensation of mild pressure and lightheadedness. Brain fog that comes and goes based on sleep quality and activity levels is more likely to be a normal postpartum symptom than the type that persists or worsens over time, which may instead signal a deeper issue. See chapter 13 for help keeping brain fog from getting out of control.

Irritability and Mood Changes

A wide range of emotions is normal and expected in the postpartum period. From exuberant joy because of your family's new addition to mourning the loss of how things used to be, layered and complex emotions are part of the human experience. However, recurrent or persistent negative feelings, particularly those that worsen over time, signal the likelihood of something deeper. While most OB and midwife offices screen for depression at postpartum visits, symptoms like irritability, anxiety, or dramatic changes in emotions are often missed by mental health screenings of this nature even though they can be just as debilitating. Mood changes are also more likely to be a health concern when accompanied by other symptoms and patterns of symptoms. We will address these in part 2. See chapter 13 for strategies for preventing mood swings postpartum.

Menstrual Changes

In the first few weeks postpartum, women experience a loss of blood and fluid from the uterus called lochia, which is not the same as a menstrual period. However, for some women—especially those who do not nurse or pump—menstrual periods return within a few weeks. The first few periods may not occur at regular intervals and may differ from your prepregnancy periods. This is normal. However, by the third period, trends should emerge, and your symptoms and experiences will likely reflect your new normal. Periods that are very heavy or light, very frequent or sparse, or accompanied by pain, clotting, or other symptoms for several months in a row are not likely to be the consequence of normally shifting hormones in the postpartum period and may reflect a deeper issue. See part 2 to understand what might contribute to these abnormalities.

At-Home Treatment for Normal Menstrual Changes (Breastfeeding-Safe)

- **Dandelion root tea:** Dandelion root extract reduces oxidative stress on the liver and improves detoxification and elimination.[7] Drinking one to three cups of organic dandelion root tea naturally supports these cleansing pathways.
- **Cruciferous vegetables:** These are a natural source of estrogen-detoxifying chemicals.[8] Consuming a half-cup serving of cooked cruciferous vegetables daily offers up to 150 g of detox-supporting Diindolylmethane (DIM) to regulate estrogen metabolism. It's important to consume the vegetables cooked, as the heat exposure increases DIM content sixfold.[9]
- **Saunas:** Sauna use promotes detoxification through sweating and the movement of lymph to eliminate metabolic waste and prevent hormonal imbalances.

Recurrent Fevers

Fevers are a sign of an immune-mediated inflammatory response and should not normally occur postpartum. The presence of a fever, particularly a high fever over 101 degrees Fahrenheit, is a sign of a problem, and you should make an appointment with your healthcare provider right away, particularly if you are still bleeding after birth or have unhealed wounds. Fever with or without pain may also point to autoimmunity (see part 2), malignancy, or a tissue infection, especially in breastfeeding mothers.

Breast Pain

Resulting from shifting hormone levels and tissue growth, breast tenderness is common both during pregnancy and in the first few weeks afterward. Breasts and nipples may also become sore due to milk production. However, breastfeeding should not be painful, and any normal discomfort would be both mild and short-lived. Persistent breast pain, or pain accompanied by fevers, nipple retraction, lumps, skin changes, or bloody discharge is a sign of a deeper, underlying problem, such as infection or malignancy, and should be evaluated by a specialist right away. Less serious causes include sex hormone imbalances as well as the conditions outlined in part 2.

At-Home Treatment for Normal Breast Pain (Breastfeeding-Safe)

- **Cold compress:** Application of a cold compress reduces swelling and inflammation of tissues, relieving pain.
- **Gentle massage:** Light massage that gently moves tissue and fluid from the nipple toward the chest wall helps clear inflammation and lymph. Use a light touch, as too much pressure may worsen swelling and pain.

- **Reverse-pressure softening (engorgement):** Pain and tenderness that result from normal breastfeeding engorgement, occurring during the early days of breastfeeding or throughout the weaning process, can be improved by gently pressing four fingers (two on either side of the nipple) toward the chest wall for a few minutes.
- **Evening primrose oil:** Supplementation with this herbal oil extract has been shown to reduce breast pain associated with hormonal fluctuations. Studies also show that it relieves the pain associated with Raynaud's phenomenon of the nipple, a blanching and reduction in blood flow that occasionally occurs in nursing mothers.[10] Dosage ranges from 2,000 mg to 4,000 mg daily.
- **Iodine:** Supplementation with molecular iodine reduces breast pain associated with hormonal changes in women when dosed at either 3 mg or 6 mg daily,[11] though in my clinical experience, much lower dosages are often just as effective. Please be aware that iodine supplementation of this nature is not safe if you have certain types of thyroid disease. Iodine supplementation may take up to three months to relieve pain.

Dry Skin and Rashes

In the postpartum period, dry skin commonly results from skin shrinkage that accompanies weight loss. Typically, it is no more severe than what frequent handwashing or dry winter air would cause, and it can easily be remedied by drinking water. Note that the nutrition strategies outlined in chapter 13 are also important for maintaining supple, well-hydrated skin postpartum. However, severe or persistent dry or itchy skin, especially if accompanied by redness, rashes, flaking, or hives is never normal. These skin conditions—including psoriasis and eczema—may be triggered by postpartum hormonal shifts. Autoimmune disorders, thyroid disease, and insulin resistance may also show up on the skin with accompanying changes in color, texture, and discomfort.

At-Home Treatment for Dry Skin (Breastfeeding-Safe)

- **Deep moisturizers:** Topical application reduces itching and redness associated with dry skin. I recommend that my patients use creams containing 1 percent colloidal oatmeal and saccharomyces ferment medium (or ferment filtrate) as an antioxidant and anti-inflammatory.
- **Evening primrose oil:** This herbal oil extract has been demonstrated to reduce dryness of skin and improve firmness and elasticity when dosed at 1,500 mg daily.[12] It also helps improve eczema.[13]

Pelvic Changes

Whether delivering a baby vaginally or via C-section, the body undergoes significant changes to structure and function. While pressure and pulling sensations are a normal experience postpartum, pelvic pain is not—whether that be during sexual activity, urination, bowel movements, exercise, laughing, sneezing, or any other time. Neither is leakage, even though it may seem like a rite of passage. Even persistent bloating or bulging of the abdomen may be a sign of dysfunctional changes to the pelvic floor that warrant rehabilitation. In addition to mechanical reasons, pelvic changes following pregnancy may result from pelvic organ prolapse, fibroids, ovarian cysts, and even endometriosis. In part 2, we will address pelvic floor dysfunction more comprehensively. General stretching and strengthening exercises are outlined in chapter 13.

At-Home Treatment for Normal Pelvic Changes (Breastfeeding-Safe)

- **Pelvic floor therapy:** I always recommend making a preventive appointment with a pelvic floor physical therapist as soon as possible after delivery.
- **Magnesium lotion:** It is normal and expected to feel like you ran a marathon after giving birth. Application of lotions containing magnesium relaxes sore and tight muscles, relieving tension and promoting sleep, especially when used before bed.
- **Bathroom ergonomics:** If you've ever heard of a Squatty Potty and don't already use one, postpartum is definitely the time to start. A seated squatting position gently relaxes stretched, bruised, and sore muscles to improve elimination. Avoid prolonged sitting on the toilet, which can strain the pelvic floor. Apart from during bowel movements, I recommend keeping knees together while sitting (including while nursing) to help the pelvic floor heal and tighten appropriately.

Weight Changes

We live in a culture that is overly critical of changes in women's bodies. Many of us hold the unrealistic expectation that our bodies will return to exactly the way they looked before conceiving, despite the fact that the pelvis permanently widens, abdominal muscles separate, breasts grow, and skin stretches through the process of pregnancy and childbirth. In the postpartum period specifically, essential rest leads to (often temporary) loss of muscle and changing metabolic expenditures that may lead to weight changes for some women. This is normal. However, dramatic and progressive weight gain or loss, particularly when it cannot be explained by changes to nutrition and exercise patterns, or when it is accompanied by other symptoms, may signal a shift in hormones or other aspects of health. Utilize the strategies outlined in chapter 13 to help your body naturally regulate weight balance postpartum.

Acne

I often say in my practice that pregnancy is like going through puberty in nine months, and childbirth is like going through puberty in one day. Postpartum hormonal shifts are swift and dramatic, and such intense fluctuations commonly trigger skin changes. However, symptoms of postpartum, including the potential for small spots of acne, should be temporary and relatively minor. New onset of or persistent acne that does not clear up after the first few weeks postpartum more likely results from an underlying health problem.

At-Home Treatment for Acne (Breastfeeding-Safe)

- **Low-tox skin products:** Beauty and hygiene products may clog pores or cause inflammation. Choose products that are free of phthalates, parabens, and sodium lauryl sulfate. I also recommend browsing the

Environmental Working Group's "Skin Deep" database for certified products that are less likely to impact skin negatively.[14] Consider unscented tallow-based moisturizers and soaps, which are gentler on skin.

- **Cruciferous vegetables:** Cruciferous vegetables contain biochemicals that naturally detoxify inflammatory estrogens, a common cause of acne.[15] Consuming a half-cup serving of cooked cruciferous vegetables daily is a great way to prevent and control postpartum acne.
- **Ozonated olive oil:** This oxygen-rich oil disrupts the cellular membrane of acne-causing bacteria and stimulates the parts of the immune system responsible for repairing skin. Also useful in control of eczema and psoriasis, sparsely applied ozonated olive oil works wonderfully for spot-treatment of postpartum acne. Please note that it is not recommended to be used as a preventive treatment or daily moisturizer.[16]

Hot Flashes and Night Sweats

As in menopause, steep drops in estrogen levels that occur during postpartum may trigger periods of intense heat sensations, which may or may not be accompanied by sweating. Night sweats occur primarily during sleep and are typically accompanied by drenching sweat. In normal circumstances, flushing does not persist beyond the first week or two of the postpartum period. If it worsens over time or lasts beyond the early days, have this symptom thoroughly evaluated, as it may be a sign of malignancy or other conditions outlined in part 2. Nutritional and stress support strategies can be very effective in managing hot flashes. See chapter 13 for details.

At-Home Treatment for Hot Flashes (Breastfeeding-Safe)

- **Maca root (*Lepidium meyenii*):** Studies have demonstrated that maca is an effective herbal remedy for reducing the frequency and severity of hormonally driven hot flashes when dosed at 1,000 mg twice daily.[17] The E-lactation database categorizes maca as very low risk for breastfeeding mothers,[18] and its historical use as a foodstuff also speaks to its safety when used by nursing mothers.

Constipation

The progesterone levels of pregnancy and structural changes that result from delivering a baby often wreak havoc on the digestive system. For this reason, many obstetricians and midwives prescribe stool softeners and laxatives postpartum to alleviate constipation. While these may ease bowel movements in the early postpartum period, they should not be needed for more than a few days. Persistent constipation, particularly the sort that lasts several weeks or longer, is likely to be the result of another underlying health condition.

At-Home Treatment for Constipation (Breastfeeding-Safe)

- **Magnesium:** Supplementation with up to 400 mg of magnesium citrate or oxide is safe for most people to use long-term to alleviate constipation.
- **Ginger:** Ginger is a gas-relieving herb that stimulates bowel movements without acting as a laxative when dosed at 1,200 mg per day.[19]

- **Bathroom posture:** A seated squatting position relaxes sore and bruised pelvic muscles to allow easier passage of stool. Consider using a Squatty Potty or other bathroom stool when voiding or during bowel movements.
- **Water and fiber:** Nutrition and hydration are essential for gut health. See chapter 13 for details on how to use nutrition to prevent constipation postpartum.
- **"I love you" massage:** Gentle manipulation of the abdominal organs also increases bowel motility and can stimulate bowel movements. (Please note that this technique is not appropriate in the early weeks following a C-section.) To perform an "I love you" massage, apply gentle pressure with your fingertips into the upper left quadrant of the abdomen, below the ribs, and slide fingertips straight down toward the left lower quadrant, as if you were drawing the capital letter *I*. Next, starting in the upper right quadrant, apply pressure moving across the abdomen from right to left, and then pivot 90 degrees to move down toward the left lower quadrant, as if drawing a capital letter *L*. Finally, beginning in the right lower quadrant, apply pressure in an upside-down U shape, moving up toward the ribs, across the abdomen, and ending in the left lower quadrant. This series of I-L-U motions traces the path of the colon and can help relax the body to stimulate bowel movements.

Headaches

Most of us have headaches from time to time. However, the stress, sleeplessness, and hormonal shifts of postpartum may temporarily increase frequency or severity of headaches without causing concern. That being said, persistent headaches, those that are particularly severe or that come more frequently than ever before, are red-flag signs that need to be evaluated. In rare cases, they may even be a sign of an emergency situation such as an infection, blood clot, stroke, neurological reaction to epidural anesthesia, or postpartum preeclampsia. Water, sleep, nutrition, and hydration are essential for preventing the most common types of postpartum headaches. See chapter 13 for details.

At-Home Treatment for Headaches (Breastfeeding-Safe)

- **Omega-3 fatty acids:** Research shows that taking 1,500 mg daily of EPA and DHA omega-3 fatty acids effectively prevents some types of migraine headaches.[20]
- **Curcumin:** When used as a preventive against headaches, twice-daily supplementation of 500 mg curcumin (a turmeric derivative) reduces frequency and severity of headaches.[21]

Changes in Milk Supply

While milk supply and composition do normally change throughout the postpartum days, even beyond the transition from colostrum to full milk, some changes are not normal. For example, a declining milk supply that leads to poor weight gain in the baby, a sudden drop or increase in milk supply that occurs several months postpartum, or other breastfeeding changes may signal a hormonal or metabolic problem. Note that in some cases return of menstruation triggers a temporary cyclic drop in milk supply. While this is not necessarily pathological, it may affect the baby's weight gain, depending on whether or not they are getting additional calories from solid food.

At-Home Treatment for Changes in Milk Supply (Breastfeeding-Safe)

- **Eat when the baby eats, drink when the baby drinks:** In my experience, postpartum mothers tend to underestimate their nutritional and hydration needs. See chapter 13 for more strategies to support breastfeeding through nutrition.
- **Ensure proper pump flange fitting:** Just as not all breasts are the same size, pump flanges are not one-size-fits-all. If you are pumping, check your flange fit and size during pregnancy, within a few days postpartum after your milk comes in, and again at six weeks postpartum. Breast size and flange fitting can fluctuate, even throughout the day. I also recommend avoiding hands-free pumps and pumping bras because they are not as efficient at removing milk as hands-on pumping techniques. Over time, poor milk extraction from breasts can lead to a permanent drop in supply.

Dizziness

The hormonal shifts of postpartum often trigger lightheadedness. Dizziness that persists or that worsens over time is unlikely to be the result of a normal process and needs to be evaluated clinically. See chapter 13 for strategies to prevent dizziness in the postpartum period. In addition to the conditions outlined in part 2 of this book, dizziness may also result from blood clots, postpartum preeclampsia, infection, migraines, or even allergies, which may develop for the first time or worsen in the postpartum period.

A Gentle Reminder

Over the course of the postpartum experience, it's normal to feel different than you did before giving birth. You will never be quite the same physically, emotionally, or spiritually. But there does come a point when postpartum symptoms stop being normal and instead signify a problem that needs, at the very minimum, to be evaluated by a healthcare provider. Although I do not by any means want to suggest that every little symptom might be a sign of a health crisis, it's important to recognize that postpartum can, and often does, trigger health problems. I don't want you to assume that debilitating symptoms you experience are "just part of becoming a parent." You deserve to feel your very best so you can enjoy your baby and your life.

My call to you as this chapter comes to a close is to trust your gut. If you are experiencing new symptoms and you don't like how you feel, get it checked out. Make an appointment sooner than your regularly scheduled six-week postpartum visit or ask for an additional appointment if that visit doesn't sufficiently address your concerns. Let the knowledge of these symptoms empower you to take your health into your own hands, whether by supporting your well-being at home or by bringing it to an office setting with full knowledge of what you need your doctor to address. You are the expert on you!

PART 2

Getting Practical

Diagnosing and Treating Postpartum Health Conditions

When advocating for your health in the postpartum period, it helps not only to know what your symptoms are but also to have a general understanding of what might be going on if your experience reflects a deeper health problem. That's what part 2 of this book is all about—giving you a better idea of when normal crosses over into becoming abnormal.

Consider the two following scenarios.

Scenario One

Doctor: "What brings you in today?"

Patient: "I have been experiencing hair loss, and I'm worried it will continue."

Doctor: "Hair loss is common in the first three months postpartum and can continue for up to a year. It results from shifting hormones that affect how hair sheds during and after pregnancy. Postpartum hair loss won't last forever, and the hair you lose will regrow. Don't worry! We can revisit it in a few months if you're still worried about it then."

Scenario Two

Doctor: "What brings you in today?"

Patient: "I have been experiencing hair loss, and I'm worried it will continue. I have done some research and some of my other symptoms have made me concerned that something deeper is going on."

Doctor: "Hair loss is common postpartum, but tell me—what are your other symptoms?"

Patient: "I've also been experiencing fatigue, body aches, and weight changes. I feel very swollen and have been struggling with constipation. I know that many of these symptoms may be a normal part of postpartum, but I understand that they may also result from nutrient deficiencies or thyroid disorders, which are commonly triggered by childbirth. Can we please take an in-depth look at my vitamin levels and thyroid function?"

In both scenarios, well-meaning doctors try to understand the patient's symptoms and provide support. However, because the postpartum symptoms referenced are so common, it's easy for the doctor to assume they're related to a recent pregnancy and delivery. But just because childbirth may be a cause of the symptoms, it doesn't mean that something else can't be. Unlike in the first scenario, the patient in the second one is armed with the knowledge that the other symptoms she is experiencing, despite also being part of a normal postpartum experience, combine to create a pattern that may point to a deeper issue, like a thyroid disorder. This knowledge empowers her to ensure that the problem is addressed thoroughly early on, without allowing a potentially serious problem to fester for several months before revisiting.

Using This Section of the Book

Now that we know what is and isn't normal postpartum, it's time to dive into the details of what drives postpartum health problems and how to fix them. This section will address seven conditions that are commonly triggered postpartum. In addition to exploring how these health conditions produce symptoms that may commonly be mistaken as a normal part of the postpartum experience, for each condition we will also outline

- what each condition involves and how it develops;
- other red flags that this condition may be a concern for your health;
- the testing protocol for diagnosing the condition; and
- possible treatment options—including risks, benefits, and alternatives.

If you suspect that you are dealing with one or more of these conditions, write down your concerns to bring to your next doctor's appointment.

Let's get started!

Health Screening Questionnaire

What differentiates normal postpartum from *not* normal? This is the big underlying question when considering a new mother's health experience. As we outlined in chapter 4, many women experience some or all of a set of common symptoms after delivering their babies. That is, at least for a while. However, if these symptoms persist, or if they are present at a heightened level of severity, they may signal a problem that needs to be checked out.

However, the symptoms outlined in chapter 4 are not the only symptoms of autoimmune disease, thyroid disorders, or other health conditions often faced by new mothers. Sometimes these seemingly normal symptoms are accompanied by other clinical signs that, when combined with a few of the expected experiences (e.g., weight changes or fatigue), create a suspicious pattern. In taking a closer look at these patterns, it often becomes clear that despite their ubiquity in the postpartum period, things like hair loss or joint pain are not normal and instead point to a bigger problem. That's what this questionnaire is here for.

Under each health condition category, you will find a list of symptoms commonly experienced by those dealing with the given problem. Keep in mind that while some symptoms are present in both the normal list and the problem lists, any of the symptoms discussed in chapter 4 could truly be abnormal, especially if part of a larger pattern. Please also remember that while a list of symptoms is not diagnostic of a given health condition on its own, these patterns of symptoms alert you that such health conditions could be a possibility for you. As you work through these checklists, take notes and make an appointment to discuss any concerns with your doctor.

Please note that not everyone experiencing the health conditions outlined in this book (or any other health concerns) shares the same symptoms, and some may not have any symptoms at all. Furthermore, the symptoms listed in any given category may signal an entirely different problem than the one described. For this reason, I recommend a health screening of all postpartum women, including those who are asymptomatic, to identify and treat problems early. Please be in communication with your healthcare providers to establish a plan for testing, diagnosis, treatment, and to share any and all health concerns. This questionnaire is an educational tool designed to raise awareness and is not intended to replace the care of a licensed healthcare provider.

How to Use This Questionnaire

Before beginning this questionnaire, take a moment to reflect on your health. Consider if there are any areas in which you do not feel satisfied with your physical or mental well-being. Note these areas before proceeding with the questionnaire.

When you're ready, read through the list of symptoms in each category. Place a check mark next to each item that resonates with you. If you find yourself checking off several items under each column in addition to one or more of the potentially normal symptoms, it could be a sign that you may be dealing with that health condition. At the bottom of each list, you'll find a chapter reference for where you can go to learn more about that disease or disorder, including what it is, which treatment options exist, and how to talk to your doctor about testing you for it.

Please also be aware that it's possible to have any of the conditions outlined in this book even without symptoms beyond what might otherwise be considered normal or even without having any symptoms at all. Furthermore, some of the conditions outlined in part 2 of this book do not classically carry additional symptoms beyond those considered to be a normal part of postpartum, such as omega-3 fatty acid deficiency (which often brings symptoms of dry, flaky skin or brittle hair or hair loss, all of which could possibly be considered normal). This doesn't make them *truly* normal but does highlight the fact that the postpartum symptoms in the "potentially normal" category are by no means exclusive to normal experiences.

Curating Your "Differential Diagnosis" List

When a healthcare provider evaluates a patient, part of the diagnostic workup involves making a "differential diagnosis" list. This consists of all the possible conditions that *may* be causing a patient's symptoms, which the doctor then uses to inform the types of tests that they order. In this book, for the sake of not letting anything slip through the cracks for your health, I'd encourage you to consider all of your symptoms as worth evaluating, regardless of whether or not they could be considered normal.

As you work your way through the questionnaire, you may find that you are placing more check marks in certain categories than others. This is how you might narrow down your own differential diagnosis list to get a clearer picture of what is the most likely culprit behind your symptoms. While it's certainly possible that any of these conditions (or more) are responsible for your health experiences, the categories with lots of check marks are the ones that you should rank at the top of your list. Use your differential diagnosis list to inform conversations with your healthcare providers.

"Normal" Postpartum Symptoms (Which May or May Not Actually Be "Normal")

Depending on the circumstances, it's possible for any of the symptoms in this list to be considered normal. However, given that they are also often symptoms of all the health conditions outlined in part 2 of this book, I would encourage you to evaluate them through a critical lens to make sure that you don't accidentally overlook something that could be an important flag for your health. Take special note if you mark any of the same symptoms in the other categories in addition to what you find on the "normal" postpartum checklist below.

Postpartum Symptoms

- ☐ Aches and pains (body aches and joint pain)
- ☐ Acne
- ☐ Brain fog
- ☐ Breast pain
- ☐ Constipation
- ☐ Dry skin or rashes
- ☐ Fatigue
- ☐ Hair loss
- ☐ Headaches
- ☐ Hot flashes or night sweats
- ☐ Insomnia
- ☐ Irritability and mood changes
- ☐ Menstrual changes
- ☐ Numbness/tingling and swelling
- ☐ Pelvic changes
- ☐ Recurrent fevers
- ☐ Weight changes

Symptoms of Iron Deficiency

- ☐ Anxiety or feelings of panic
- ☐ Body aches and pains
- ☐ Brain fog
- ☐ Breathlessness
- ☐ Cravings for nonfood items, especially dirt, ice, or metal
- ☐ Dizziness

- ☐ Fatigue
- ☐ Hair loss
- ☐ Headaches
- ☐ Heart palpitations
- ☐ Irritability
- ☐ Menstrual changes
- ☐ Pale or dry skin
- ☐ Racing heart
- ☐ Sore or swollen tongue

See chapter 5, "Nutritional Deficiencies"

Symptoms of Vitamin B_{12} and/or Folate Deficiency

- ☐ Appetite changes
- ☐ Brain fog
- ☐ Breathlessness
- ☐ Fatigue and muscle weakness
- ☐ Indigestion
- ☐ Loose stools
- ☐ Mood changes
- ☐ Mouth sores/swollen tongue/burning mouth
- ☐ Numbness/tingling in hands and feet
- ☐ Pale skin
- ☐ Racing heart
- ☐ Slow wound healing
- ☐ Vision changes
- ☐ Weight loss

See chapter 5, "Nutritional Deficiencies"

Symptoms of Zinc Deficiency

- □ Brain fog
- □ Brittle or discolored nails
- □ Frequent illness
- □ Hair loss
- □ Mood changes
- □ Neurological problems
- □ Sensitive skin
- □ Thyroid or adrenal disorders

See chapter 5, "Nutritional Deficiencies"

Symptoms of Vitamin D Deficiency

- □ Brain fog
- □ Dry skin
- □ Fatigue
- □ Frequent illness
- □ Headaches
- □ Mood changes
- □ Pale skin

See chapter 5, "Nutritional Deficiencies"

Symptoms of Omega-3 Fatty Acid Deficiency

- □ Dry skin or rashes
- □ Hair loss

- ☐ Headaches
- ☐ Mood changes
- ☐ Slow wound healing

See chapter 5, "Nutritional Deficiencies"

Symptoms of Hypothyroidism (Including Hashimoto's Disease and Postpartum Thyroiditis)

- ☐ Constipation
- ☐ Depression or other mood changes
- ☐ Difficulty swallowing
- ☐ Dry skin
- ☐ Fatigue
- ☐ Feeling too cold
- ☐ Goiter (swollen thyroid)
- ☐ Hair loss
- ☐ Heavy or irregular menstrual periods (if returned)
- ☐ Hoarse voice
- ☐ Infertility
- ☐ Low blood pressure
- ☐ Muscle weakness
- ☐ Puffy face
- ☐ Slowed heart rate
- ☐ Unintentional weight gain

See chapter 6, "Thyroid Disorders"

Symptoms of Hyperthyroidism (Including Graves' Disease and Postpartum Thyroiditis)

- ☐ Anxiety
- ☐ Fast or irregular heartbeat, palpitations
- ☐ Goiter (swollen thyroid)
- ☐ Hyperactivity
- ☐ Increased blood pressure or heart rate
- ☐ Increased sweating
- ☐ Insomnia
- ☐ Loose stools
- ☐ Menstrual changes
- ☐ Sensitivity to heat
- ☐ Swelling around eyes
- ☐ Unintentional weight loss

See chapter 6, "Thyroid Disorders"

Symptoms of Autoimmune Disease (Including Thyroid Autoimmunity, Rheumatoid Arthritis, and Systemic Lupus Erythematosus)

- ☐ Brain fog
- ☐ Dizziness
- ☐ Fatigue
- ☐ Joint pain
- ☐ Mood changes
- ☐ Recurrent low-grade fever

- ☐ Recurrent miscarriage
- ☐ Swollen glands or joints

See chapter 7, "Autoimmunity"

Symptoms of Autoimmune Bowel Disease (Including Celiac Disease, Crohn's Disease, and Ulcerative Colitis)

- ☐ Abdominal pain
- ☐ Black, tarry stools
- ☐ Bloating and gas
- ☐ Bowel urgency or incontinence
- ☐ Constipation or diarrhea
- ☐ Dry skin or rashes
- ☐ Fatigue
- ☐ Fevers of unexplained origin
- ☐ Hair loss
- ☐ Joint pain or stiffness
- ☐ Mouth ulcers
- ☐ Nausea or vomiting
- ☐ Osteoporosis
- ☐ Rectal bleeding
- ☐ Recurrent miscarriage
- ☐ Weight changes

See chapter 7, "Autoimmunity"

Symptoms of Multiple Sclerosis

- ☐ Brain fog
- ☐ Dizziness or vertigo
- ☐ Fatigue
- ☐ Numbness or tingling in arms or legs
- ☐ Poor coordination
- ☐ Tremors or muscle spasms
- ☐ Vision changes

See chapter 7, "Autoimmunity"

Symptoms of Psoriasis

- ☐ Brittle nails
- ☐ Fatigue
- ☐ Hair loss
- ☐ Joint pain
- ☐ Rashes
- ☐ Small dents in nails

See chapter 7, "Autoimmunity"

Symptoms of Adrenal Dysfunction

- ☐ Abdominal pain
- ☐ Body aches
- ☐ Brain fog
- ☐ Constipation or diarrhea
- ☐ Cravings for salt or sugar

- ☐ Dizziness
- ☐ Fatigue
- ☐ Hair loss
- ☐ Increased sweating
- ☐ Irregular periods (if returned)
- ☐ Low blood pressure
- ☐ Mood changes
- ☐ Nausea
- ☐ Palpitations
- ☐ Recurrent illness
- ☐ Sensitivity to light, sound, or other stimulation
- ☐ Skin tags
- ☐ Weight changes

See chapter 8, "Adrenal Dysfunction"

Symptoms of Insulin Resistance

- ☐ Difficulty losing weight
- ☐ Discolored or darkened skin patches (particularly in skin folds, groin, or armpit)
- ☐ Dry skin or rashes
- ☐ Fatigue, especially following meals
- ☐ Frequent yeast infections
- ☐ Gout
- ☐ Increased appetite or sugar cravings
- ☐ Increased thirst
- ☐ Skin tags

See chapter 9, "Insulin Resistance"

Symptoms of Pelvic Floor Dysfunction

- ☐ Constipation
- ☐ Frequent need to urinate (including overnight)
- ☐ Frequent urinary tract infections
- ☐ Heaviness or pressure in vagina and/or vulva
- ☐ Hernia
- ☐ Inability to achieve orgasm
- ☐ Leakage of urine or stool
- ☐ Low back pain
- ☐ Pelvic pain, including pain with sex
- ☐ Progressively worsening varicose veins in vulva or legs
- ☐ Visible bulging at the vaginal opening

See chapter 10, “Pelvic Floor Dysfunction”

CHAPTER 5

Nutritional Deficiencies

Have you ever heard the phrase "eating for two"? While it would be nice for the nutritional needs of pregnancy and lactation to be as simple as doubling portions of usual meals and snacks, pregnancy requires both more and less than that at the same time. The same goes for breastfeeding, a nutritionally demanding process that involves converting everything from cheeseburgers to chopped salads into perfectly balanced milk to feed another human. But whether or not you can or choose to breastfeed, the incredible demands of pregnancy itself mean that the baby's health sometimes comes at the expense of the mother's. I often joke that the sacrifices of motherhood start in the womb, as our bodies put the baby's well-being above our own, ensuring that our child has access to the zinc, B vitamins, iron, and fatty acids that they need, even if doing so requires subtracting from our body's own stores (much less replenishing our losses).

Resources abound for prenatal nutrition, but what all of them have in common is the fact that none of them is specific to *you*, *your baby*, or *this particular pregnancy*. (Yes, nutritional needs can change not just from mother to mother but from pregnancy to pregnancy!) While our bodies often give us guidance through cravings and overall increased hunger, it's still easy for nutritional deficiencies to develop because we don't all have access to (or the desire to eat) perfectly nutritious food all the time. Not to mention, many women experience severe food aversions or nausea and vomiting (so called morning sickness) during pregnancy, which can lead to deficiencies despite our best intentions. Many women, because of the growing size of the baby, also struggle to consume enough food late in the third trimester without feeling too full. It's not uncommon, actually, for late-third-trimester mamas to plateau in their weight or even lose weight despite the baby's growth. Then, when we factor in pregnancies with multiples, you can see how the nutritional math gets very complicated very quickly.

While all nutrients are needed at somewhat heightened levels during pregnancy, some of the key nutrient deficiencies I see in postpartum patients that produce symptoms that mimic "expected" postpartum symptoms include:

- iron
- vitamin B_{12}
- folate
- zinc
- vitamin D
- omega-3 fatty acids

Unfortunately, because there is no standard screening protocol for postpartum women, preventive testing for nutrient deficiencies is not typical. Providers may test for iron deficiency in women who experienced profound blood loss during delivery, or if some of the more severe neurological symptoms related to vitamin B_{12} deficiency show up, for example. However, in my experience, obstetric providers are unlikely to test for deficiencies of zinc, folate, vitamin D, or omega-3s, even if many of the symptoms occur. I routinely run these labs for postpartum patients, and these nutrient deficiencies are very common. Everyone should be screened for them! Let's discuss how these deficiencies produce symptoms, what those symptoms look and feel like, and how you can talk to your doctor about testing for them postpartum.

Iron

Strange though it may seem, the very same iron that we need to consume in our diets is used to make wrought iron fences and cast-iron pans. Our bodies convert that metal into hemoglobin, a protein found inside red blood cells, which carries oxygen everywhere that it needs to go. Oxygen provides cellular energy, so not getting enough iron means not getting enough oxygen and consequently having symptoms like depleted energy and a slowing down of all the systems that need energy to function. In other words, nothing works properly in our bodies when iron levels drop. Women with iron deficiency experience profound fatigue, different from sleepiness or wanting to rest after a busy day. Anemic patients describe it as having had their batteries taken out, like their muscles don't want to work, and that their bodies feel heavy and slow.

Now, all new moms know that the sleep deprivation wrought by newborn interruptions is also a "different kind of tired." So, we can't differentiate iron deficiency from sleep deprivation or other types of expected postpartum exhaustion based on feeling tired alone. Looking at other symptoms of iron deficiency and the timing of their onset helps discern the culprit behind fatigue. That being said, if you have any suspicions at all about your health, get it checked out! The challenge of sifting through symptoms is precisely the reason I recommend testing iron levels in all postpartum women as part of a preventive screening program.

Symptoms of Iron Deficiency

Because iron—and oxygen—are required for the function of every cell in the body, the potential symptoms range just as widely. However, here are a few of the most common that I see, which doctors often mistake for normal:

- fatigue
- pale skin
- hair loss
- brain fog
- dizziness
- breathlessness
- heart palpitations or the sensation of a racing heart
- sore or swollen tongue
- anxiety and panic attacks
- pica, a phenomenon involving cravings for nonfood items such as dirt, ice, or metal (you may or may not actually consume these items)

Iron deficiency often develops because of a diet lacking iron-rich foods such as spinach, beans, red meat, and poultry. However, it also commonly develops during pregnancy because of increased nutritional demands and a rapidly expanding blood supply. Iron deficiency in pregnancy is pretty common, and symptoms of it frequently start before delivery. Think back in time: If your symptoms started before your little one joined you earth side, you may be dealing with deficiency of iron or other nutrients.

Blood loss during delivery also commonly causes iron-deficiency anemia. When it comes to timing, this is the most challenging to discern—blood loss, the physical exertion of labor, and newborn sleep interruptions all start at roughly the same time: your baby's birthday! If you find that you don't feel any better by a few days past delivery, after you've recovered a bit from the physical work involved in childbirth, consider this a red flag for iron deficiency.

In relatively rarer cases, postpartum inflammation or new onset of autoimmune disease also leads to iron deficiency. In these situations, the fatigue may creep up more slowly, and you might realize that you actually felt *better* immediately after delivery than you feel a few months out. Iron deficiency and autoimmunity can both develop at any time postpartum. Make an appointment to get labs done, and take a look at chapter 7 to learn more about autoimmune disease.

Testing for Iron Deficiency

- **Complete blood count (CBC):** This panel measures red blood cell (RBC) parameters, like total red blood cell count and size, as well as hemoglobin and hematocrit, which reflect iron content of RBCs. Prolonged iron deficiency impairs production of healthy RBCs, and blood loss decreases total RBC numbers.

- **Serum iron:** This reflects the level of iron in your bloodstream at any given time, which fluctuates depending on absorption ability, recent dietary patterns, and supplementation.
- **Total iron binding capacity (TIBC):** Apart from red blood cells, a type of protein called transferrin carries iron molecules in the blood. Think of these transferrin proteins as city buses. A high TIBC means there are a lot of empty seats on the bus and not enough iron molecules to fill them.
- **Percent saturation:** Another way of measuring the transferrin-iron relationship, this test reflects the percentage of occupied seats on the transferrin city bus.
- **Ferritin:** This measures the body's iron stores. Whereas other tests such as serum iron fluctuate more quickly, ferritin gives a bigger picture—an understanding of the body's iron reserves.

Treatment for Iron Deficiency

Correcting the problem of iron deficiency may seem obvious—consume more iron. While in severe cases a blood transfusion or iron infusion may be required to correct iron deficiency, nutritional strategies and supplementation sufficiently address the problem in most cases.

When it comes to iron-rich foods, not all sources are created equal. Even though the same iron our bodies need can be found in wrought iron fences and iron pipes, these metal objects do not employ iron the same way our red blood cells do. In other words, elemental iron of this nature is not as biologically available. Our bodies absorb and utilize iron from animals, who themselves metabolize iron into biologically active forms much more easily than plants do. Additionally, plants naturally contain other compounds, like calcium and tannins, which inhibit absorption of iron from these foods. Because of this, I recommend prioritizing consumption of red meat like grass-fed (ideally also grass-finished) beef as well as quality, cage-free eggs. I certainly also encourage you to eat salads and hummus, but when it comes to harnessing the power of food to correct iron deficiency, animal sources work tremendously well, and plants simply don't.

The same holds true for correcting iron deficiency through supplementation. In addition to inferior absorption, most over-the-counter iron supplements are harsh on the gut, causing symptoms like nausea and constipation. My best recommendation for those who need supplementation is heme-based iron, derived from porcine or bovine sources. These products offer superior absorbability with minimized risk of side effects.[1] If you prefer an elemental supplement, iron bisglycinate is less likely to cause constipation than iron sulfate. Iron supplements should be taken on an empty stomach, and all at once rather than in divided doses, to reduce gastrointestinal side effects. Alternatively, these supplements can be taken with a small amount of a vitamin C–rich food or a vitamin C tablet to improve absorption.

Vitamin B12 and Folate

Iron isn't the only nutrient that causes fatigue when levels drop. Whereas iron carries oxygen and energy to our cells, vitamin B_{12} plays a key role in helping us turn food into energy. Metabolism and energy production are some of the most important and well-known functions of vitamin B_{12} in the human body.

Meanwhile, vitamin B_{12} and other B vitamins like folate (vitamin B_9) are also involved in numerous other processes that our health depends on, such as the making of red blood cells. In our discussions of iron, we explored the important ways that red blood cells carry oxygen to all of our bodily tissues. Vitamin B_{12} and folate are required to form healthy, mature red blood cells that are capable of carrying oxygen in the first place. Synthesis of DNA—the genetic code telling our bodies how to grow and function—also depends on these nutrients. All aspects of cellular repair and regeneration require DNA, which therefore means they require folate and vitamin B_{12} too. Additionally, B vitamins help detoxify our bodies, protect our brains and neurons, and regulate our mood via neurotransmitters.

When our bodies don't have enough vitamin B_{12}, we experience symptoms like mood changes, vision changes, fatigue and muscle weakness, brain fog or poor memory, and numbness or tingling in our hands and feet. Deficiency of folate, like B_{12}, may also contribute to slow wound healing, pale skin, loose stools, indigestion, breathlessness, mouth sores, and a swollen tongue. Some people describe the sensation of a burning mouth with deficiency of folate or B_{12}. Even digestive problems, appetite changes, weight loss, and a racing heart may result from not getting enough vitamin B_{12} or folate.

These deficiencies usually develop from a diet that does not sufficiently sustain the demands of pregnancy and, if applicable, breastfeeding. Any combination of symptoms provides enough reason to ask your doctor for B_{12} and folate testing, but timing of these symptoms also provides clues: Dietary deficiency that starts during pregnancy means symptoms likely also start before the baby is born. Likewise, symptoms that come on after a few weeks or months of breastfeeding may signal depletion patterns.

Dietary Sources of Vitamin B_{12} and Folate

Liver from cows and chickens is one of the best dietary sources of both B_{12} and folate. If you don't like to eat organ meat, you still need to eat animals. Meaningful quantities of vitamin B_{12} can only be found in foods of animal origin, unless food manufacturers add synthetic forms to their products through fortification.[2] Meanwhile, the best food sources of folate (outside of liver) are leafy green vegetables and legumes.

Some digestive disorders, including celiac disease, ulcerative colitis, and Crohn's disease, affect absorption of vitamin B_{12} and folate, which damages the receptors responsible for uptake of these nutrients in the small intestine. Vitamin B_{12} deficiency may also develop from pernicious anemia, an autoimmune condition affecting the stomach and small intestine. Certain medications also affect absorption of these nutrients. Metformin (prescribed for gestational diabetes), H2 receptor blockers, and proton-pump inhibitors (prescribed for heartburn) affect vitamin B_{12} absorption,[3] while drugs used in the treatment of certain autoimmune and inflammatory conditions (sulfasalazine, methotrexate) as well as certain antibiotics and seizure medications interfere with the body's ability to absorb and utilize folate.

Please note that genetic mutations affecting the enzyme methylenetetrahydrofolate reductase (MTHFR) may also lead to impaired utilization of folate, with profound health implications. The testing and treatment of MTHFR mutations is beyond the scope of this book, but please note that these mutations should be suspected and tested for in all individuals with folate-associated signs, symptoms, or disorders, as well as in mothers of children born with neural tube defects.

Testing for Vitamin B_{12} Deficiency

- **Vitamin B_{12}:** This is the simplest and most obvious way to test B_{12} levels. While lab ranges may vary, it is widely accepted that a patient should be further evaluated for B_{12} deficiency if serum levels are below 400 pg/mL, even if above the laboratory minimum.[4]
- **Folate:** This is the simplest and most obvious way to test for folate deficiency. However, it's also important for another reason; because folate and B_{12} are both involved in the development of red blood cells, folate sometimes corrects the RBC problems caused by low B_{12} (see below). However, because folate doesn't substitute for all functions (especially neurological ones), folate supplementation may accidentally mask a deficiency of B_{12}, leading to misdiagnosis. Prenatal vitamins are very high in folate, so postpartum women are particularly at risk of this misdiagnosis pattern. It's important to test for both vitamin B_{12} and folate when patients have symptoms of deficiency, even with normal red blood cell markers.
- **Complete blood count (CBC):** Deficiency of B_{12} or folate may lead to red blood cells of an increased size

(mean corpuscular volume, aka MCV), as well as low hemoglobin, hematocrit, or red blood cell count.

- **Bilirubin:** Red blood cells that form improperly due to B_{12} or folate deficiency break down at a higher-than-normal rate, elevating blood levels of bilirubin.
- **Lactate dehydrogenase (LDH):** Like bilirubin, LDH levels elevate when red blood cells break down rapidly due to B_{12} or folate deficiency.
- **Methylmalonic acid (MMA):** Deficiency of vitamin B_{12} causes blood levels of MMA to build up. High levels signal a B_{12} deficiency, often before CBC markers change. This is considered the most sensitive test for B_{12} deficiency.
- **Homocysteine:** Similar to MMA, deficiencies of vitamin B_{12} or folate cause homocysteine levels to rise in the blood, signaling the possibility of deficiency.

Treatment for Vitamin B_{12} Deficiency

The most obvious treatment for deficiency of B_{12} and folate is to ensure adequate dietary intake through whole food forms and to supplement when necessary. I recommend a diet rich in high-quality animal products, including fish, shellfish, poultry, and meat for vitamin B_{12}, as well as green vegetables for folate. Liver and eggs are excellent sources of both.

With supplementation, not all forms are equal. Folic acid (the synthetic form of folate) and cyanocobalamin (the synthetic form of vitamin B_{12}) are common in fortified foods and supplements. However, neither of these lab-derived products is the metabolically active form that can be used by the human body. Instead, it's a better choice to supplement with 5-methyltetrahydrofolate for folate[5] and either methylcobalamin or adenosylcobalamin for vitamin B_{12}.[6] In cases of profound deficiency or impaired digestive absorption due to intestinal disease, injections of vitamin B_{12} or folate may be required.

Zinc

Like iron, zinc is another metal that our bodies require for proper functioning. Known as the hair, skin, and nails mineral,[7] zinc also helps the body with energy utilization, immunity, making new DNA molecules, and producing thyroid,[8] adrenal,[9] and sex hormones.[10]

Zinc deficiency affects every system that uses it, potentially leading to abnormal immune system function, thyroid and adrenal disorders, poor quality skin and nails, hair loss, brain fog, mood changes, neurological problems, impaired sense of taste and smell, and frequent illness. The most common cause of zinc deficiency is insufficient dietary intake. The nutritional demands of pregnancy and breastfeeding[11] as well as digestive disorders and medications like proton-pump inhibitors that decrease absorption (typically prescribed for heartburn) may also lead to deficiency.

Testing for Zinc Deficiency

- **Zinc serum:** This test measures zinc in the bloodstream, which fluctuates relatively easily. Low levels indicate deficiency, but normal levels may not mean that the body has adequate zinc stores.
- **Zinc, RBC:** Red blood cells survive about three months before breaking down. Red blood cell levels

of zinc therefore reflect average zinc status over the previous three months and subsequently give a better indication of zinc storage. However, in the early postpartum months, mothers are still detoxifying higher blood counts from pregnancy, and this level may be artificially inflated, possibly giving a false negative for zinc deficiency.

Treatment for Zinc Deficiency

Oysters, fish, shellfish, and meat are the best dietary sources of zinc. Beans and some types of nuts also provide dietary zinc.[12] Grains like corn and rice contain phytic acid, which inhibits absorption of zinc, so those with this deficiency may consider avoiding or limiting these foods.[13] Among supplementation options, zinc picolinate is best absorbed.[14] Note that high doses of zinc, particularly above 50 mg for several weeks, may affect absorption of other nutrients and lead to another deficiency, such as copper or magnesium.[15] In my practice, I usually recommend supplementation of copper and magnesium along with zinc for this reason.

Vitamin D

What do autoimmune diseases[16] (including those affecting the thyroid[17]), fatigue,[18] cognitive impairment,[19] depression,[20] and cortisol imbalances[21] have in common? Optimal vitamin D levels reduce the risk of developing all of them.

Vitamin D functions more like a hormone,[22] traveling through the bloodstream to bind to receptors on nearly every cell of the body, even influencing gene expression.[23] For this reason, it's no surprise that nearly all the symptoms considered normal in the postpartum period may be able to be attributed to vitamin D—or lack thereof—in some capacity. This is especially true of brain fog and fatigue, mood changes, dry skin, and headaches. Vitamin D–deficient patients also report pale skin and frequent illnesses.

Vitamin D is supposed to be synthesized in the skin from UV exposure, as it is not classically a dietary vitamin. Lack of sunlight due to indoor lifestyles limits sunlight and subsequent UV exposure, leading to deficiency. This is exacerbated by well-intentioned but short-sighted recommendations to avoid the sun for fear of sunburn and increased skin cancer risk. Unfortunately, evidence also suggests that exposure to environmental toxins such as air pollution[24] and pesticides[25] interferes with vitamin D production pathways in human skin and is another meaningful contributor to the epidemic of vitamin D deficiency. Researchers in epidemiology currently estimate that 35 percent of US adults are deficient in vitamin D,[26] with levels less than 30 ng/mL, though many experts agree that optimal levels actually range between 40 and 70 ng/mL.[27] Using that standard, a far greater proportion of us are probably deficient too.

Testing for Vitamin D Deficiency

- **25-OH vitamin D:** This test measures total blood levels of vitamin D.

Treatment for Vitamin D Deficiency

Vitamin D blood tests evaluate total levels of vitamin D_2 and D_3, two different forms of this micronutrient. However, when supplementing to correct deficiency, vitamin D_3 is more effective at raising and restoring blood levels.[28] Because vitamin D is a fat-soluble vitamin, it is possible to overdose on it. I recommend working with a healthcare provider to monitor blood levels when supplementing. Look for a supplement that also contains a small amount of vitamin K_2, as this combination works synergistically to improve effectiveness and reduce risks.[29]

Perhaps you are wondering about sunlight (UVB) exposure as a preventive or treatment for vitamin D deficiency. Indeed, this is the most biologically normative means for getting vitamin D. However, because the UV index varies so widely according to latitude, season, cloud cover, and time of day, there is no good rule of thumb for the optimal "dose" or time required for sun exposure. Furthermore, skin type influences the amount of vitamin D produced in any given person, and vitamin D metabolism varies from person to person as well. Researchers studying this question published a proposed model that states that exposing one-third of the whole body to one-third of the amount of sunlight that would be required to cause sunburn at noon (the period of most direct sunlight) during a warm sub-period of the year in low- and midlatitude regions (for example, between April and September in the southern United States) provides approximately the equivalent level of vitamin D to 2,000 IU taken orally.[30] I don't know about you, but I didn't have the gumption for such convoluted math problems when I was postpartum!

Instead of trying to predict something so difficult, I typically recommend that my patients supplement with enough vitamin D to bring their blood levels back up to normal, and at the same time suggest that they spend as much time outside as they can without getting sunburned. We then monitor their levels of vitamin D via bloodwork over the course of time to see if their outdoor habits are sufficient to decrease or wean off oral supplementation with vitamin D. Generally speaking, because of our modern lifestyles and responsibilities, this isn't usually possible. Maintaining optimal levels through sun exposure alone is really tough, especially in the winter months or for those who live up north. Vitamin D is one of those things that I end up recommending my patients continue to supplement long-term.

Omega-3 Fatty Acids

Not all fats are the same. There are "good fats," like olive oil, "bad fats," like hydrogenated shortening, and what I would call "exceptionally beneficial fats," like omega-3s. We normally talk about omega-3s in terms of their benefits to heart health, but they also play a major structural role in the brain and nervous system,[31] help control the immune system and inflammation (including that which drives autoimmunity),[32] regulate reproductive[33] and adrenal hormones,[34] and have been proven as a treatment for some types of depression.[35]

Because of the recommendation that pregnant and breastfeeding women limit consumption of seafood,[36] compounded by the prevalence of more pro-inflammatory omega-6 fatty acids in American processed foods, many postpartum women lack sufficient levels of omega-3 fatty acids and experience negative health implications as a result. These include increased risk or worsening of inflammatory and hormonal disorders, many of which are triggered for the first time postpartum. Individuals deficient in omega-3 fatty acids also report dry skin, rashes, brittle hair or hair loss, mood changes, and even headaches.

Testing for Omega-3 Deficiency

- **OmegaCheck:** This test measures levels and proportions of omega-3 and omega-6 fatty acids, the types of fat that we tend to consume in excess due to ultra-processing of foods and ubiquity of seed oils, which displaces our intake of omega-3s.

Treatment for Omega-3 Deficiency

The single best way to correct an omega-3 deficiency for the long-term is to regularly consume foods rich in them. While both plant and animal foods contain omega-3s, the only plants that offer two of the most important omega-3s—EPA and DHA—in meaningful amounts are algae and seaweed, which most people don't consume abundantly enough to maintain adequate fatty acid intake. Instead, I recommend eating high-quality, low-toxin fatty fish, such as sardines, four or five days per week.[37] Alternatively, you can consider supplementing with a high-quality omega-3 fish oil or krill oil. Algae-based DHA supplements are also an option for those affected by fish allergies.

CHAPTER 6

Thyroid Disorders

I shared my own experience with finding out I had postpartum thyroiditis at the beginning of this book. Thyroiditis is so common in postpartum women that it has its own special name. However, it is by no means the only thyroid condition that can be triggered, flare, or otherwise be present for the first time after pregnancy and childbirth. Anyone who has been pregnant knows that it is not just a condition of the reproductive system; it affects the whole body. Growing an entire new human (or humans) requires a tremendous amount of energy and nutrition, and the thyroid sets the thermostat for all these processes of growth, development, and energy utilization. At the same time, the thyroid gland is the subject of some of the most common autoimmune conditions. These are of particular concern in the prenatal and postpartum periods due to the dramatic ways that pregnancy affects the immune system. In this chapter, we'll dive into the details of the most common thyroid disorders postpartum women face. This will include autoimmune thyroid disorders, but please note that we will cover the additional autoimmune conditions triggered by pregnancy in the next chapter.

Identifying Thyroid Problems

Perhaps you are reading this section because you suspect you have a thyroid problem, maybe even based on symptoms identified in the health questionnaire provided at the beginning of part 2. Then again, maybe you are simply curious if you should talk to your doctor about screening for a thyroid disorder, or you want to know what treatment options might look like if you do find out about a new diagnosis. The main thing you need to know is that despite a prevalence of thyroid issues among women, there is currently no recommended standard screening for thyroid disorders postpartum.[1] (In my practice, thyroid problems rank highest on my list of suspicions for pretty much any postpartum symptom.) Because of the lack of screening standardization, your doctor will probably not test you for thyroid disorders following pregnancy unless they have a reason to. Therefore, if you want a thorough thyroid workup after giving birth, you need to either

1. directly ask for screening and explain your reasoning for wanting it (i.e., your cause for suspicion, family history, personal history), or
2. bring relevant symptoms to your provider's attention so they can connect the dots and test what needs to be tested.

Types of Thyroid Disorders

Thyroid dysfunction develops for many reasons and may come on at any time in life. Notably for the purpose of this book, some types of thyroid disorders are more common following pregnancy and childbirth and are understood to be directly triggered by the hormonal and immunological shifts involved. Knowledge of these conditions will help you know what to ask your doctor about when it comes to screening and postpartum visits. Bear in mind that a person does not need to have all the given symptoms for a diagnosis to be made, and some women even have no symptoms at all. Here's an overview of the main categories of thyroid disorders that are most relevant to women who recently gave birth:

- **Hypothyroidism** refers to the state of having an underactive thyroid, meaning metabolic processes slow down. In hypothyroid disorders, many patients experience symptoms like fatigue and weakness, depression, hair loss, unintentional weight gain, low heart rate, low blood pressure, constipation, dry skin, cold intolerance, facial puffiness, irregular periods, infertility, and more. Because of the possible development of a goiter (a swollen thyroid), many patients also develop vocal hoarseness or difficulty swallowing. Causes of new-onset hypothyroidism include but are not limited to the hormonal shifts associated with pregnancy, infections, autoimmunity (such as Hashimoto's thyroiditis), toxin exposure, nutrient deficiencies, postpartum blood loss, and postpartum thyroiditis.

- **Hyperthyroidism** refers to the state of having an overactive thyroid, meaning that metabolic processes speed up. In hyperthyroid disorders, many patients experience symptoms like anxiety, insomnia, heart palpitations, unintentional weight loss, loose stools, heat intolerance, excessive sweating, hyperactivity, and increased blood pressure or heart rate. Some patients even experience tremors and swelling around their eyes or neck swelling (goiter). Still others have no symptoms at all. Causes of new-onset hyperthyroidism include but are not limited to the hormonal shifts associated with pregnancy, autoimmunity (such as Graves' disease), viral exposures, excess consumption of iodine, use of certain medications, and postpartum thyroiditis.
- **Autoimmune thyroid disease** encompasses several underlying causes of thyroid inflammation, which comes from the body's self-defense response. Autoimmune thyroid disease may be triggered by immune system shifts that occur during pregnancy, infections, trauma, and toxin exposure, among other reasons. Even in patients with normal thyroid function, those with autoimmune thyroid disorders often also experience fatigue, joint pain, depression, obsessive-compulsive symptoms, and problems with memory or focus.[2] It may also be accompanied by recurrent low-grade fevers of unexplained origin, joint pain and muscle aches, dizziness, and fertility problems. Note: Autoimmune thyroid disease may or may not result in hyper- or hypothyroidism and produces symptoms on

its own because of the inflammation involved. These symptoms may overlap with the conditions of hyperthyroidism or hypothyroidism but also may not.

- **Postpartum thyroiditis** refers to a condition of thyroid inflammation and dysfunction occurring within twelve months of pregnancy for those who had normal thyroid function prior to conception. This includes both pregnancies that ended early in miscarriage or termination as well as those that ended in full-term delivery. Postpartum thyroiditis often begins with a state of hyperthyroidism, followed by hypothyroidism, and then, in some cases, ends with spontaneous resolution of thyroid dysfunction. An estimated 20 to 40 percent of women remain hypothyroid long-term following postpartum thyroiditis.[3] Postpartum thyroiditis has a strong relationship with autoimmune thyroid disease.

Testing for Thyroid Disorders

When it comes to thyroid testing, most doctors do a pretty good job of running thyroid screening tests when the patient's symptoms call for it. However, another big problem in the care of not just postpartum women but of patients in general is that the basic thyroid screenings performed are not sensitive enough to identify the full breadth of thyroid problems that may occur. In many ways, the standard screening does not even sufficiently identify the *most common* thyroid condition! Let me explain.

To test a patient's thyroid function, some or all of the following tests may be used. How and when these tests are run tends to depend on the provider and what they're looking for in the patient. Let's take a look at what they are:

- **Thyroid-stimulating hormone (TSH):** This is the simplest and most common thyroid screening test. TSH is produced in the brain, enters the bloodstream, and stimulates the thyroid to produce thyroid hormones.
- **Free T4:** This is the second most common piece of a thyroid screening test. When stimulated by TSH, the thyroid produces this hormone, which makes up the vast majority of all thyroid hormone produced.
- **Free T3:** Once the thyroid makes T4, it travels in the bloodstream to different parts of the body, where it is then converted into T3 and used directly by cells. Because conversion of T4 to T3 depends so much on these other parts of the body, T3 is not considered to reflect thyroid function as directly—T3 levels depend on much more than just the thyroid gland. However, levels of T3 still matter in terms of how a patient feels and how their body functions.
- **Total T4:** The thyroid gland produces much more thyroid hormone than the body uses in any given moment. However, making thyroid hormones takes a substantial amount of time, and metabolic needs change more rapidly than what the thyroid can keep up with. So, it's a good idea to have a backup or storage of thyroid hormone to use more quickly when it's needed. To do this, the body makes more T4 than is needed, and the extra attaches to proteins and rides around in the bloodstream. When needed, the extra T4 hops off

the proteins and goes where it needs to go. Conditions like pregnancy, certain medications, illness, and other health changes influence the levels of these proteins, so total T4 is not accepted to be as reliable of a measure of thyroid function as free T4.

- **Total T3:** This is the equivalent of total T4 and its relationship to blood proteins, except measuring T3 instead.
- **Antithyroid peroxidase (TPO) antibodies:** This test screens for a type of antibody produced by the immune system that destroys thyroid hormone–producing enzymes. This is considered a more sensitive and specific screen for autoimmune thyroid disease.[4] It is part of the diagnostic criteria for autoimmune thyroiditis, and the vast majority of patients with Hashimoto's disease, Graves' disease, and postpartum thyroiditis test positive for anti-TPO antibodies.
- **Anti-thyroglobulin (Tg) antibodies:** This test screens for antibodies that target and damage the building block proteins involved in making thyroid hormones. It may be positive in Hashimoto's disease, Graves' disease, and postpartum thyroiditis, or may be negative in all of these conditions, depending on the individual.
- **Thyroid-stimulating immunoglobulin (TSI):** This type of antibody targets receptors on the thyroid responsible for triggering thyroid hormone production. High levels lead to increased thyroid hormone production, and the presence of this antibody is specific to Graves' disease (an autoimmune thyroid disease that causes hyperthyroidism).

Up to 18 percent of the adult population (nearly one in five) tests positive for anti-TPO and/or anti-Tg antibodies,[5] meaning that the immune systems of these patients make antibodies targeted toward proteins in the thyroid, causing inflammation, damage,[6] and the substantial risk of eventually developing thyroid disease. Most notably, women who test positive for thyroid antibodies in early pregnancy have up to a 52 percent chance of developing postpartum thyroiditis, and—get this—if they still test positive in the third trimester, the likelihood of them developing the condition spikes to 80 percent.[7] The American Thyroid Association recommends the following treatment strategies for patients with positive thyroid antibodies:[8]

- Consider levothyroxine (thyroid medication) therapy in all women using assisted reproductive techniques (like IVF and IUI) who test positive for thyroid peroxidase antibodies.
- Test TSH levels *every four weeks* from the time pregnancy is confirmed until midpregnancy in women who have normal thyroid function prior to delivery but positive thyroid antibodies.
- Use 25–50 mcg of levothyroxine in women with normal thyroid function but positive thyroid antibodies who also have a prior history of pregnancy loss.

How, though, is a woman supposed to know that she is one of the 18 percent of people who tests positive for thyroid antibodies if her providers have never tested her? Realistically, most providers simply don't test their patients for this because it is not the standard of care, whether in preconception counseling, pregnancy screenings, or postpartum. Even the standard thyroid screens don't include this important marker, instead including just TSH and free T4. I recommend that you ask your doctor for an anti-Tg and anti-TPO antibody test as a preventive screening, even if you don't have symptoms, even before you become pregnant. This is information that your future health depends on.

Treatment for Thyroid Disorders

The big question in the room when it comes to thyroid disorders is what you're supposed to do about it if you have one of these conditions. Most of the time, doctors prescribe medication for their patients when thyroid disorders are identified, but they may take a "watch and wait" approach, depending on the situation. In my practice, I often tend to recommend doing more and less at the same time. Let me explain.

Normal Thyroid Lab Tests

Thyroid hormone levels, especially for TSH, fluctuate widely throughout the day. In the case of normal thyroid labs with suspected hypothyroidism, a doctor may be quick to discount symptoms as normal if the first round of thyroid screens come back in the normal range.

Do More

- Ask for another round of testing, completed a week later, to confirm accuracy of the testing.

- Make sure your doctor also includes thyroid antibody testing in addition to the other markers on a full thyroid hormone panel. Remember that autoimmunity produces symptoms—often mimicking thyroid-related symptoms—even in the absence of thyroid hormone abnormalities.
- If those labs come back normal as well, remember that it's not normal to feel unwell, and your doctor needs to test for other health conditions if your thyroid isn't the culprit.

Do Less

- Stay off prenatal vitamins, multivitamins, or anything containing biotin for at least three days prior to testing, as this may interfere with the accuracy of the test.
- Diagnostic tests, doctors' appointments, and slow-to-come answers can be stressful. Be gentle with yourself and build in extra rest time while you get to the bottom of your health concerns.

Hypothyroidism

The typical treatment for hypothyroidism is levothyroxine (name brand: Synthroid). Many providers do not offer their patients other options and may not even be aware that other options exist.

Do More

- Add T3. Levothyroxine is a synthetic replacement for T4. However, other medications that contain both T3 and T4 exist, like Armour Thyroid, which has been shown to alleviate symptoms more effectively than levothyroxine.[9] NP Thyroid is another option containing both T3 and T4 replacement, and the medication liothyronine is a synthetic T3 prescribed as an adjunct for patients whose symptoms do not improve from levothyroxine alone.

- Make sure you find out if your hypothyroidism stems from autoimmune origins by requesting thyroid antibody testing from your doctor. Uncontrolled autoimmunity leads to progressively worsening hypothyroidism, so it's important to address the immune system too. Here's what the research says about treating patients with elevated thyroid antibodies:
    - » Selenium supplements can help calm the immune system's attack on the thyroid, both on their own and in combination with levothyroxine medication.[10] I recommend that my patients use 200 mg for at least six months, monitoring bloodwork.[11]
    - » Myoinositol improves thyroid health, especially in combination with vitamin D[12] and selenium.[13] Based on the research available, I recommend my patients supplement with at least 600 mg myoinositol.
    - » Low-dose naltrexone (LDN) is a lower prescription dosage of a drug classically prescribed in the treatment of addiction disorders. More recently, it has gained traction due to its effectiveness in treating a variety of inflammatory and autoimmune

disorders.[14] Although research regarding its use in thyroid treatment is limited, LDN is emerging in the field of functional medicine as an increasingly popular and comparatively safe treatment option for autoimmune thyroid disorders, mediated through its ability to suppress inflammatory pathways.[15]

Do Less

- Thyroid medication isn't always necessary. Research shows that eliminating exposure to thyroid-damaging toxins,[16] following a gluten-free diet,[17] and improving gut health through probiotics[18] regulate thyroid hormone production and overall thyroid function. Additionally, thyroid function worsens with poorly controlled blood sugar.[19] Talk to your doctor about addressing the other systems of your health before or in combination with starting thyroid medication.
    - » Environmental toxins impacting thyroid function include:
        - Perchlorate in contaminated drinking water, food, and fabrics[20]
        - Polychlorinated biphenyls (PCBs), dioxins, and furans in contaminated animals and seafood[21]
        - Phthalates such as those found in personal care products[22]
        - Lead in contaminated food, dust, water, and soil[23]
        - Mercury such as from eating contaminated fish[24]

Hyperthyroidism of Autoimmune Origin

The autoimmune disorder Graves' disease causes most cases of hyperthyroidism.[25] Hyperthyroid conditions caused by other factors are beyond the scope of this book. Treatment options for Graves' disease include beta-blockers, which is a class of medications commonly used for the cardiovascular symptoms associated with hyperthyroidism, as well as antithyroid drugs like methimazole (the first-line treatment in non-pregnant women) and propylthiouracil (during pregnancy). In severe cases, doctors may recommend surgical removal of the thyroid or destruction of the thyroid tissue through administration of radioactive iodine.

Do More

- L-carnitine: Review studies demonstrate the benefit of 2 g a day of L-carnitine in reducing cardiac arrythmia, thyroid storm, and other hyperthyroid symptoms. It even helps some patients reduce dependency on antithyroid medication.[26]
- Lemon balm and bugleweed: Although the research in support of these herbs is not as robust as other thyroid treatments, case studies have repeatedly demonstrated resolution of hyperthyroidism with treatment of herbal tinctures containing lemon balm and bugleweed.[27]
- Chinese medicine: Large-scale review studies have demonstrated the effectiveness of traditional Chinese medicine in treating patients with Graves' disease. While the nature of this medicine is highly individualized, research has shown promising results

with use of *Tripterygium wilfordii*, *Prunella vulgaris*, Yinjia pellet, and Yikang pill.[28]

Do Less

- Less iodine: Excessive iodine exposure is a well-documented trigger of hyperthyroidism, which is of concern in all cases of elevated thyroid function but especially Graves' disease.[29] While some iodine is still necessary for human health despite diagnosed thyroid conditions, pay attention: Are you receiving excess exposure to or consuming too much iodine, to the point that it may be affecting your thyroid function? Sources include supplements, iodized salt, and other fortified foods like bread, potatoes (sometimes grown in iodized soil), seaweed, kelp, and more.
- Less methimazole: In my clinical experience, methimazole is not always effective at eliminating symptoms of Graves' disease and its associated laboratory abnormalities. Furthermore, studies demonstrate that up to 50 percent of patients maintain remission after a twelve- to eighteen-month course of the drug versus long-term use—another common prescription strategy.[30] Talk to your doctor about a shorter course of medication or trialing elimination if the medication is not bringing about the intended effects on your health. While it's not wrong or bad to use medication, that medication should arguably fix the problem it's being taken to solve.

Postpartum Thyroiditis

While autoimmunity triggers the vast majority of postpartum thyroiditis cases, not all have this cause. If you test positive for thyroid antibodies in combination with receiving a diagnosis of postpartum thyroiditis, be sure to observe the guidelines outlined in the "Hypothyroidism" section earlier for strategies that apply to autoimmune cases.

Postpartum thyroiditis treatment often does not require medication, but in some cases may involve a short course of beta-blockers in the hyperthyroid phase and possibly thyroid hormone replacement, such as the medication levothyroxine, in the hypothyroid state.

Do More

- Because the majority of postpartum thyroiditis cases resolve without progressing to permanent hypothyroidism, many women receive no long-term thyroid follow-up after resolution.[31] Because of the risk of future thyroid disease, ask your doctor for regular, thorough thyroid screenings throughout the rest of your life.
- Up to 84 percent of women with postpartum thyroiditis relapse with subsequent pregnancies.[32] Take a proactive approach and ask for thyroid screenings during pregnancy, at two weeks postpartum, and every month for the first year.

Do Less

- Given that most cases do resolve without permanent hypothyroidism, consider talking to your doctor about weaning off or eliminating the medication under medical supervision to see how your body copes without it. Sometimes simply out of sheer inertia, women prescribed levothyroxine in the hypothyroid phase of postpartum thyroiditis remain on the drug long-term, perhaps unnecessarily.

- With any case of autoimmune thyroiditis (or autoimmunity in general) but especially in the postpartum period, stress provokes the autoimmune response. This means that women are both more sensitive to and less tolerant of stressors *on a physiological level.*[33] Take every available effort to decrease your workload, sleep as much as possible, outsource household and other tasks, and generally decrease your stress to improve your health.

CHAPTER 7

Autoimmunity

Young, old, pregnant, and otherwise immunocompromised. Time and time again, my college professors harkened back to these four groups of people because of their vulnerability and risk. I studied food science in college, and a large part of my training focused on food safety. This meant going above and beyond to prevent contamination of food products for the sake of the YOPIs—young, old, pregnant, and otherwise immunocompromised. I'm pretty sure "YOPIs" was the answer to at least one final exam question each semester. They are *that important*.

In some ways, the list of four could easily be simplified under the umbrella of immunocompromised, because that's exactly what they all have in common. The babies, the elderly, chemotherapy patients, those with HIV/AIDS or other immunodeficiencies, and—yes—pregnant women are all considered immunocompromised. Recounting our brief discussion in chapter 2, pregnant women's bodies undergo tremendous immune shifts to protect the growing baby. Despite being our own children, fetal cells are not *our own cells*, and our immune systems are programmed to reject and attack all such foreign bodies (think *streptococcus* bacteria, flu viruses, *salmonella*, etc.)—that is, unless our immune systems dampen down to allow an entirely separate human to grow within us for nearly ten months, which is exactly what happens. As a result, other things also have more of an opportunity to grow, which increases our risk of infection as well as our risk of complication from infections. Hence, we are immunocompromised.

But what happens when we deliver our babies and our immune systems remain suppressed? Or what happens when the systems rebound with a vengeance, losing the ability to distinguish between self and nonself, attacking everything from our thyroid gland to our skin to the DNA of our cells? Unfortunately, for some women this dysfunction becomes reality, and that is what we mean by autoimmunity. As it stands, women make up the majority of autoimmune sufferers—roughly 80 percent—and they have a significantly greater likelihood of contracting an autoimmune disease within twelve months of delivering a child compared to other seasons of life.[1] This risk is even higher in those who deliver via cesarean section compared to those with vaginal births, perhaps triggered by the mixing of blood during the procedure.[2] Researchers also identified increased risks of developing autoimmunity in the three years following delivery among mothers who experienced pregnancy complications, including preeclampsia, spontaneous preterm birth, and stillbirth.[3]

The immune shifts that occur during pregnancy and postpartum stretch far and wide, with many postpartum symptoms pointing directly back to immune system function or *dys*function. Even postpartum depression has been identified as having roots in autoimmunity.[4] I often say that with autoimmunity, when it rains, it pours; the presence of one autoimmune condition points to future risk of developing additional autoimmune diseases. I appreciate how researchers Syreen Goulmamine, Sarah Chew, and Irene Aninye put it in their 2024 article titled "Autoimmune Health Crisis: An Inclusive Approach to Addressing Disparities in Women in the United States." They wrote, "Thyroid autoimmunity is often considered a gateway to other autoimmune states because individuals diagnosed with more than one autoimmune disease are likely to have a thyroid autoimmune disease—either presenting clinically first or subclinical post diagnosis."[5] The first diagnosis paves the way for future autoimmune diagnoses, but in many cases, it is the pregnancy itself that opens the gate to the autoimmune path in the first place.

As if developing an autoimmune disease postpartum isn't tough enough already, it's made even worse by delayed diagnosis due to the tremendous overlap in symptoms between "normal" postpartum and an objectively not normal autoimmune condition. From fatigue to hair loss, skin changes, weight gain or loss, joint pain and stiffness, and digestive shifts, even the most well-intentioned doctor can easily miss what would seem like obvious warning signs if they presented in a different season of life. When reflecting on your own symptoms, here's a table that might be helpful in differentiating between expected postpartum symptoms and autoimmune disease.

Symptom	Normal Postpartum	Autoimmunity
FATIGUE	Generally improves over time in relationship to sleep duration and quality. Observational research has shown that most women who experience profound fatigue at ten days postpartum feel noticeable improvement by three months,[6] though the effects of sleep may take up to six years or more to fully resolve.[7]	Worsens in seemingly unpredictable flares or persists and progressively worsens with time. For those with autoimmune disease, fatigue may remain longer than expected following otherwise uncomplicated illness. A good rule of thumb is that if you aren't starting to feel better by three months or once your baby sleeps predictably, it's a good idea to see your doctor.
HAIR LOSS	Tends to start within two to four months postpartum and resolve with new hair growth between six to twelve months. Timeline may be delayed with breastfeeding and weaning.[8] Usually affects the whole scalp equally.	Starts any time and may progressively worsen, with the key differentiating factor being persistence of symptoms.[9] Autoimmune hair loss is more likely to occur with patches, scarring, or inflammatory scalp changes, but may not always.
SKIN CHANGES	Mild dryness and loss of elasticity, which may have been present during pregnancy. Researchers found that these changes tend to persist, sometimes four months postpartum or longer.[10]	May include patches of redness, flaking, blistering, peeling, profound itching, hives, or other rashes that are never normal. May occur at any time or flare following illness, sleeplessness, or stress.
JOINT PAIN/STIFFNESS	Postpartum aches and pains may be similar to joint pain experienced in pregnancy, like hip and low back pain. Research shows that more than 80 percent of postpartum women report resolution of pelvic/low back pain by six weeks, though discomfort may pop up again in places that make sense (i.e., upper back and shoulders from poor breastfeeding posture).[11] Ultimately, normal aches and pains tend to improve with time.	Tends to affect joints that aren't subject to overuse; comes in flares every few days/weeks/months and usually progressively worsens over time. Autoimmunity tends to affect joints that were unaffected during pregnancy, then flare with a vengeance postpartum or following periods of stress or illness.
DIGESTIVE COMPLAINTS	Mild constipation usually improves quickly, within a few days or weeks. Most women experience resolution by one month postpartum, though it may persist a bit longer in women who delivered via cesarean.[12] The same symptoms may have been present during pregnancy.	Pain, bloating, often loose stools or alternating constipation and diarrhea; worsens with time and may begin immediately after birth or several months postpartum. Often, but not always, accompanied by weight loss.

Functional Medicine Prevention for Autoimmune Disease

Autoimmunity is not just one thing. Our immune systems can run us ragged in many ways and through countless different mechanisms, affecting nearly every organ system in our bodies. However, inflammation is the overarching umbrella that different types of autoimmune diseases have in common. Whether affecting the joints in rheumatoid arthritis, the skin in psoriasis, or the brain in multiple sclerosis, inflammation is the common thread.

Because of this, functional medicine treatment for autoimmunity primarily targets inflammation. In addition to many of the specific herbal and supplementation strategies described in each subsequent section of this chapter, treatment and prevention through functional medicine requires the establishment of various anti-inflammatory lifestyle strategies. Many of these, such as nutrition, sleep, stress management, and exercise are outlined in chapter 13. However, some of the more specific strategies for supporting our immune systems and keeping inflammation contained might surprise you. The following approaches to reducing inflammation, in addition to the preventive strategies provided later in this book, help control autoimmune diseases and the risk of developing them in the postpartum period.

- **Breastfeeding:** There are a million and one reasons to support moms in their breastfeeding journeys. From the nutritional benefit to baby and the boost in longevity to mom, breastfeeding benefits the health of everyone involved. That being said, for many women, breastfeeding is not a walk in the park. I personally struggled with breastfeeding after my first child was born because of an undiagnosed tongue tie in my infant that caused latch problems and excruciating nipple trauma and pain for more than three weeks. I nearly gave up on several occasions until we had the tie revised through a laser procedure and we completed two months of physical therapy exercises, performed every four hours around the clock. But even after the pain was gone, breastfeeding still meant frequent feedings, recurrent bouts of mastitis and clogs, and an extremely complicated pumping process when I returned to work. I share all this because, despite the challenges, biology doesn't lie: Breastfeeding is good for you and protects your health. Research shows that moms who breastfeed enjoy a reduced risk of developing rheumatoid arthritis,[13] thyroid-related autoimmunity,[14] and multiple sclerosis.[15]

- **Dental hygiene:** Personally, I really struggled emotionally with the thought of going anywhere without my babies during the early postpartum period. Whether from anxiety, attachment, or mere biological instinct, something felt viscerally wrong to me about leaving the house without my teeny tiny baby in tow. The first such venture I made alone—going to the dentist—wasn't until my daughter was two months old. Truth be told, I didn't even make it through the whole cleaning before excusing myself to rush home, breasts engorged and leaking, to feed my inconsolably crying baby. In hindsight, we both could have waited an extra twenty minutes for the dental hygienist to finish scraping my teeth. But postpartum is as postpartum does. Why all the fuss about going to the dentist? Our oral health ties in tremendously with the health status of the rest of our bodies, including our immune systems. Research shows that patients with poor marks of oral hygiene, such as increased plaque buildup, face an increased risk of developing autoimmune disease.[16] It may be easy to overlook something as small as our teeth, especially when we're already overwhelmed, but our dental hygiene can have a tremendous effect on the rest of our well-being. Brush, floss, and make every effort to get to the dentist twice per year.

- **Avoiding alcohol:** I don't know about you, but dressing up and heading out to a wine bar was probably the last thing on my mind in the first year after giving birth to each of my kids. Instead, the extent of my "nightlife" was changing diapers, wiping spit-up, and trying not to trip over anything as I blindly navigated my bedroom in the dark (if you know, you know). Going out just wasn't something I had the gumption to do. Plus, when breastfeeding or co-sleeping, meaningful alcohol consumption really isn't recommended. But whether you're nursing or not, no matter who shares your bed, and regardless of the vibrancy of your social life, keeping alcohol use under control is well understood to play an important role in preventing the development of autoimmune disease through a dose-dependent association, including autoimmune thyroid disease, type 1 diabetes, lupus, rheumatoid arthritis, and multiple sclerosis.[17]

Testing for Autoimmunity

The paradox of treating patients is that sometimes one or more symptoms may point to a diagnosis but the lab tests don't necessarily support it. At the same time, lab testing holds the power to identify illnesses before symptoms even begin. As a functional medicine doctor, I see lab testing as one of the most valuable tools of modern medicine for this precise reason. Especially with autoimmune disease and the genetic predispositions involved, combined with the fact that actual onset tends to be slow, early identification is crucial for preserving your quality of life. That means that *screening tests* are an essential piece of quality care and should be part of every postpartum follow-up plan. In this section, I'll outline and explain the autoimmune screening tests that I recommend postpartum for every woman. Then, in subsequent sections, I'll detail specific diagnoses and make note of additional tests you might want to ask your doctor to run.

Once you've identified a subset of symptoms pointing to the possibility of autoimmunity, I recommend talking to your doctor about running the following labs as a screen:

- **Anti-TPO and anti-Tg antibodies:** As explained in the previous chapter, these tests screen for Hashimoto's disease but may also be positive in Graves' disease and postpartum thyroiditis, which has autoimmune origins.
- **TSI:** This is a test specifically for Graves' disease, one of the most common autoimmune conditions triggered postpartum.
- **Antinuclear antibodies (ANA) with titer and pattern:** Antibodies that target the nucleus of cells (where

the DNA is stored) highly correlate with autoimmune diseases affecting multiple organ systems, especially systemic lupus erythematosus. Rarely, cases of postpartum thyroiditis may bring mild elevations in ANA levels.[18] In the broader medical community, doctors diagnose autoimmune disease based on a combination of ANA and follow-up tests, plus a patient's physical signs and symptoms. In functional medicine, however, we recognize that it is never normal to make antibodies against one's own cells and tissues. Additionally, medical research has demonstrated that an autoimmune diagnosis is more likely to be made among younger women with symptoms of autoimmune disease and high platelet counts[19] (that remain elevated up to four weeks postpartum).[20] Unsurprisingly, the combination of these signs and symptoms closely mirror those of "normal" postpartum.

- **Rheumatoid factor:** This antibody test is positive in the majority of patients with rheumatoid arthritis.
- **C-reactive protein (CRP):** I noted earlier that the inflammation marker CRP is not a good marker for detecting postpartum health conditions because it normally remains elevated in postpartum women, sometimes for several weeks.[21] However, I wanted to include it on this list because many doctors use CRP as a screen despite the fact that it may yield false positives early on and because persistent elevations that continue to rise throughout the postpartum period also raise a red flag. Use this information to open conversation with your doctor about all the possible root causes of your symptoms.

Types of Autoimmunity and Typical Treatments

Because the immune system is interwoven with nearly every aspect of our health, the potential types of autoimmunity range just as widely. That being said, some autoimmune diseases remain extremely rare, including in the high-risk postpartum period. The following list of autoimmune diseases reflects the most common conditions triggered by pregnancy and childbirth, apart from thyroid autoimmunity,[22] with symptoms commonly mistaken to be normal.

Celiac Disease

Triggered by gluten consumption, patients with celiac disease mount an immune response targeting the lining of the small intestine. Classic symptoms include weight loss, abdominal pain, loose stools, bloating, and fatigue. However, most adults also demonstrate so-called nonclassic symptoms, including anemia, osteoporosis, elevated liver enzymes, and recurrent miscarriage, among others.[23] In my practice, I commonly see patients with skin rashes, hair loss, joint pain, anxiety, or depression, which turn out to have origins in celiac disease and its associated inflammation.

- Testing for celiac disease involves a screening blood test for IgA anti-tissue transglutaminase antibody (TG2-IgA), possibly followed by intestinal biopsy and/or IgA anti-endomysial antibody (EMA), but the patient must be eating gluten to avoid false negatives for these tests. If someone is already following a gluten-free diet, genetic testing for celiac disease utilizing HLA typing for DQ2 and DQ8 alleles can be used.[24] Typically, endoscopy with intestinal biopsy is recommended to confirm celiac disease when it is suspected. However, I always suggest treatment for anyone with positive results for TG2-IgA or EMA tests or with abnormal HLA-typing, even if biopsy results are negative. This is because many celiac sufferers present with the previously mentioned "non-classic" symptoms, which respond well to treatment, even in the absence of intestinal damage.

- Treatment involves adherence to an extremely strict gluten-free diet, and, from the perspective of functional medicine, additional strategies to support gut healing, such as supplementation of arginine, glutamate and glutamine,[25] probiotics,[26] digestive enzymes,[27] and more.

Crohn's Disease and Ulcerative Colitis

Crohn's disease (CD) and ulcerative colitis (UC) are two main inflammatory bowel diseases that are classically understood as autoimmune in nature and involve symptoms such as low back pain, abdominal pain, bloating, changes in stools, intestinal bleeding (to be differentiated from the common postpartum condition of hemorrhoids), fatigue, weight changes, joint pain, skin rashes, and fevers.

- Testing for CD and UC involves intestinal biopsy, but screening tests performed beforehand often demonstrate abnormalities on CBC panels, as well as with CRP and erythrocyte sedimentation rate (ESR). Doctors may also run stool tests for fecal calprotectin, lactoferrin, and occult blood.

- Treatment for UC usually begins with sulfasalazine and other aminosalicylates, anti-inflammatory drugs administered either orally or rectally, with biologics—medications made from or extracted from a biological source, such as cells, blood, or genes—recommended for more severe cases.[28] Crohn's disease treatment usually begins with corticosteroids, and if needed, medications that suppress the immune system. Surgery may be required for treatment of severe cases.[29] Functional medicine treatment involves probiotic therapy (especially utilization of *Bifidobacterium* strains),[30] sodium butyrate,[31] and herbal strategies including indigo naturalis,[32] deglycyrrhizinated licorice,[33] and curcumin,[34] among others.

Rheumatoid Arthritis and Systemic Lupus Erythematosus

While certainly not the only ANA-positive autoimmune diseases, rheumatoid arthritis (RA) and systemic lupus erythematosus (SLE) both bring symptoms that closely mimic normal postpartum experiences. Both conditions include joint pain and stiffness, rashes, fatigue, weight changes, and possibly fevers. Primarily affecting joints, RA involves destruction of bone and cartilage by the immune system but also may lead to lung and cardiovascular disease. In addition to skin and joints, lupus also affects kidneys, red blood cells, and the cardiovascular system.

- Testing for RA involves ANA, RF, anti-cyclic citrullinated peptide antibodies, and x-ray imaging of joints to evaluate bone changes. Diagnosis of SLE involves

ANA, anti–double stranded DNA, complement proteins, and other blood tests to evaluate organ function.

- Treatment for RA typically begins with methotrexate, which cannot be taken during pregnancy.[35] Other treatments for both RA[36] and lupus[37] may involve hydroxychloroquine, steroids, immunosuppressants, and biologic drugs. Through a functional medicine paradigm, many providers also prescribe naturally occurring compounds in supplement form, such as N-acetyl cysteine (NAC),[38] proteolytic enzymes,[39] curcumin, and liposomal glutathione[40] in treatment of RA and SLE. These natural strategies help reduce or avoid the need for prescription medications (and the side effects they bring).

Multiple Sclerosis

Multiple sclerosis (MS) is an autoimmune disease characterized by nervous system degeneration. Symptoms include extreme fatigue, muscle weakness, numbness and tingling in the extremities, problems with balance and coordination, dizziness, tremors, and cognitive dysfunction (brain fog), among others.

- Testing includes MRI imaging of the brain and spinal cord in combination with a physical exam. Samples of cerebrospinal fluid may also be collected and tested as part of the diagnostic process.
- Treatment traditionally includes drugs like interferons, glatiramer acetate, teriflunomide, fumarates, monoclonal antibodies, and biologic medications.[41] Functional

medicine also offers evidence-backed strategies to prevent decline and improve neurological function in MS patients, such as high-dose omega-3 fatty acids,[42] *Andrographis*,[43] *Boswellia*,[44] and CBD oil,[45] among others.

Psoriasis

Commonly known for its chronic, recurrent skin inflammation caused by attacks from your body's immune system, psoriasis may also affect joints, causing a unique form of arthritis. Psoriasis classically causes red patches of skin with silvery scales, most commonly on the scalp, elbows, knees, and low back. It also may affect palms of hands, soles of feet, nails, and even genitalia. But though those are the visible symptoms, psoriasis affects the whole body and often brings fatigue as an accompanying symptom.

- Testing officially relies on skin biopsy, but hallmark clinical signs and symptoms often point to the diagnosis in an office setting. X-ray imaging is involved in the diagnosis of psoriatic arthritis.
- Treatment usually involves topical steroids and calcineurin inhibitors, but doctors may prescribe methotrexate, cyclosporine, and immunosuppressants (or related drugs) in severe cases.[46] Functional medicine treatments include topical application of indigo naturalis[47] and *Mahonia aquifolium*,[48] topical or oral curcumin,[49] and combination prebiotic/probiotic therapy.[50] My patients have also benefited from topical use of ozonated olive oil, which is also profoundly helpful in controlling eczema in both infants and adults.

CHAPTER 8

Adrenal Dysfunction

Let's talk about ice cream. Ice cream is probably one of my favorite foods, and it's definitely my favorite dessert. Maybe it's yours too. However, if you've ever overindulged, you probably remember the nauseous, bloated, oversugared feeling that comes from *too much* ice cream. I certainly do, and because of this, I usually limit myself to a single scoop instead of ordering the ever-tempting double stack on a sprinkle-covered, chocolate-dipped waffle cone when my family visits ice cream shops. Out of wisdom, we restrict ourselves because we know that it's possible to have too much of a good thing. On the flip side, a world without any ice cream at all would be rather depressing—so let's just agree that we surely need *some* ice cream to support an overall sense of well-being and pleasure in life.

Of course, I'm joking (kind of), as we don't truly need ice cream to survive and thrive. But a little sugar does seem to make life sweeter.

Unlike sugar, which we technically don't *need* if we're honest with ourselves, we do need something else that gets a bad reputation: cortisol. Commonly known as the stress hormone, you might have heard warnings about the dangers of high cortisol, the risks associated with stress, and the need to keep this hormone under control. While it's true that physical, psychological, and mental stress all potentially lead to increased cortisol production and that too much cortisol harms our health, we do need *some* cortisol—just like we need all our other hormones—for our bodies to function correctly. Like ice cream, too much cortisol can harm our health, but again, like ice cream, too little affects us negatively as well. Cortisol benefits us by helping regulate our nervous systems and control our blood sugar and blood pressure, among countless other essential functions. It influences our metabolisms and immune systems, controls our sleep-wake cycles and inflammation levels, and overall supports our bodies' systems of balance.

Ice cream and cortisol also have a relationship to time in common. Just as it makes more sense metabolically to enjoy a sundae after dinner instead of first thing in the morning, there's a healthy and appropriate time of day for cortisol to be high (morning) and, likewise, an appropriate time for it to be low (evening). This is true regardless of the stressors in life, like work demands, relationship conflicts, financial constraints, parenting, and household responsibilities. Despite the dynamic nature of our lives, our bodies were designed to regulate our cortisol output according to the clock regardless of our other circumstances. That is, when everything functions as it should.

But, living in a broken world, we know that things don't always work the right way. Just like our thyroid hormones, our immune systems, and the nutritional status of our bodies, our stress hormone regulation systems change dramatically during pregnancy and don't always recover the way we expect them to postpartum. Following the hormone shifts of pregnancy and childbirth, our bodies' production and use of cortisol can fall into disruption. This produces often debilitating symptoms that, incidentally, often mimic a "normal" postpartum experience. For many of my patients struggling with hair loss, weight changes, mood swings, gut problems, fatigue, and sleep disruptions, diagnostic testing shows that their hypothalamic-pituitary-adrenal axis (HPA axis)—the technical term for the body's stress-regulation system or *adrenal system*—has fallen into disarray. While many of these patients feel frustrated and alarmed when they realize just how long a treatable problem has been left to fester, they find hope and reassurance in the fact that help and healing will come. The same is true for you, mama. Perhaps you and your doctor have tested for and ruled out nutritional deficiencies, thyroid disorders, and autoimmunity. Adrenal dysfunction could be the culprit behind your postpartum symptoms.

The Hypothalamic-Pituitary-Adrenal Axis

The *hypothalamic-pituitary-adrenal axis* is basically a fancy term for how our brains regulate our stress responses. The hypothalamus and pituitary gland together make up part of the brain's control center, regulating most bodily functions. In addition to the HPA axis, we also have an HPO (ovarian) axis and an HPT (thyroid) axis, all three of which reciprocally interact with each other to coordinate hormonal activities in the body. The HPA and other axes aren't something we can control—our brains run in the background, making decisions about everything from metabolic rate to fertility, sleep timing, and stress tolerance. In most cases, acute stress tends to set off alarm bells in these centers of the brain, impacting the signals sent to the thyroid, ovaries, and adrenal glands. This is part of the reason why women experience amenorrhea—the absence of menstrual periods—during seasons of emotional stress, from the nutritional and hormonal demands of breastfeeding, because of sleep disruptions, or on account of other taxing circumstances. While fertility may be the last thing on your mind postpartum, it's not just reproductive function that stress impacts. These same triggers also can lead to changes in thyroid function and cortisol metabolism, triggering significant symptoms.

Our bodily production of cortisol fluctuates hour by hour and minute by minute. In doing so, the cortisol circulates through our bloodstream, interacts with cells, and then gets cleared away. If we didn't metabolize cortisol in this way, the near-constant production of it would lead to exponentially rising levels throughout our lives. As a means of maintaining the status quo, our bodies try to match the rate of cortisol clearance with the rate of production, varying our production of this hormone according to our bodies' need for it throughout the day. In a well-adapted system, we'd make more cortisol during periods of stress with an accompanying increase in clearance rate, sort of like a bathtub draining at the same rate that the faucet fills it up. This process gets a little murky postpartum, though, between normal hormone shifts and the stress caused by childbirth, sleeplessness, parenting, and any of the other myriad things that can go wrong.

Pregnancy itself brings meaningful increases in cortisol production to support the baby's growth, up to even triple the normal levels.[1] Immediately following delivery of the placenta, however, cortisol production plummets, while cortisol metabolism maintains its rate. (Think: Someone shut off the faucet, but the bathtub is still draining.) In time, the rate of cortisol metabolism should normalize to match the drop in cortisol production, usually within twelve weeks. However, research shows that some women, particularly those who experience chronic stress during pregnancy, are more likely to experience a delay in the return to normal, leading to increased risk of mood disturbances, fatigue, and even thyroiditis or other autoimmune conditions, such as those discussed in chapter 7.[2] If you notice symptoms of any of the stages of HPA axis dysfunction discussed on the following pages that don't resolve by twelve weeks postpartum, you definitely need a thorough medical workup. (But mama—if you're experiencing debilitating symptoms presenting before that point, it's worth looking into for the sake of your and your baby's health.)

Disruptions in the HPA Axis

If you've ever been told that your symptoms are the result of stress, it might feel like a minimization. Sometimes the "You're stressed" type of health assessment seems to be saying "You just need to relax," or "It's all in your head," or "This is a mind over matter situation." While stress certainly can be a trigger for HPA axis dysfunction, it's not "just stress," and the symptoms that arise because of it definitely aren't all in your head. They're in your hair loss, your weight fluctuations, your irritability, anxiety, or depression. They also show up as debilitating fatigue, brain fog, body aches, recurrent illness, increased sweating, skin tags, tummy troubles, cravings, menstrual problems, changes in blood pressure, dizziness, palpitations, or feelings of overwhelm. They are a hormonal imbalance, sometimes triggered by stress, manifesting in cortisol regulation but also potentially in autoimmune disorders, thyroid problems, or future fertility concerns.

The type of stress that triggers HPA axis dysfunction comes in many forms. It may show up simply because the placenta leaves your body, or it may be related to past or current trauma. Mama, if your symptoms started following a tumultuous fertility journey, an unexpected early delivery or surgical intervention, severe illness during pregnancy, separation from your baby, NICU time, loss, colic, or any other traumatizing experience surrounding you becoming a mother, your health can be helped and your stress relieved. Most importantly, you are loved and seen, and you are not alone. Keep going.

All that being said, I have also seen HPA axis dysfunction brought on by chronically interrupted sleep from babies who themselves simply *don't*, from calorie deprivation (tip: Eat when your baby eats), returning to exercise too soon, and even infectious illness. Here are the three stages of HPA axis dysfunction:

Stage 1 HPA Axis Dysfunction—"Alarm"

During the normal stress response, the HPA axis triggers the release of cortisol, an energizing, motivating, provocative hormone that increases blood pressure, blood sugar, and attention. However, under periods of acute stress, the constant influx of cortisol transforms energy, mental focus, and motivation into anxiety, irritability, and insomnia.[3] Over time, this also leads to blood sugar dysregulation, abdominal fat gain, and loss of bone and muscle.

- Testing for Stage 1 HPA axis dysfunction uses a six-point salivary cortisol test. Stage 1 will reveal multiple samples of higher-than-normal cortisol levels throughout a twenty-four-hour period.

Stage 2 HPA Axis Dysfunction—"Resistance"

It goes without saying that chronic exposure to stress is not good for us, and the body knows it. When stressors persist, our bodies adapt in response to protect themselves from physical breakdown. In this stage, the same exposures paradoxically produce less of a total stress response, between elevated rates of cortisol clearance and decreased cortisol production.[4] This stage brings brain fog, irritability,[5] and rapidly fluctuating energy levels.

- Testing for Stage 2 HPA axis dysfunction also uses a six-point salivary cortisol test. Stage 2 results will reveal elevated morning cortisol that rapidly drops off to deficient levels later in the day. Or the tests may paradoxically reveal lower-than-normal morning cortisol with elevated afternoon or evening tests.[6]

Stage 3 HPA Axis Dysfunction—"Exhaustion"

Finally, after enough time exposed to stress and sufficient depletion of resources, our bodies enter a point of exhaustion, weakening the immune system and leading to mental and physical burnout, fatigue, mental health changes, and depleted stress tolerance.[7]

- Testing for Stage 3 HPA axis dysfunction using a six-point salivary cortisol test will reveal deficient cortisol levels along all or most points of the cortisol curve.[8]

The Root Cause of HPA Axis Dysfunction

The common denominator among all three stages of HPA axis dysfunction is exposure to stress. The longer it sticks around, the more the problem worsens, bringing with it accompanying symptoms of increasing severity. As may seem obvious, the very best treatment for the problem of HPA axis dysfunction is to identify the source of stress. However, as a new mom, it's not always easy to pinpoint where, exactly, the stress stems from.

Shortly after my second child turned one, when I had two toddlers aged two and under, a conversation with a family member highlighted to me that, once again, I wasn't okay. As a person who likes to feel generally in control and collected, works in the field of functional medicine, and identifies as someone of overall good health, I felt frustrated by the realization that I was again dealing with postpartum health challenges. At that point in life, my irritability, brain fog, inattentiveness, and fatigue were getting in the way of my ability to engage meaningfully in relationships I valued. Reluctant as I was to admit I was dealing with anything more than the need to resolve a communication error in a relationship that was important to me, I'd also learned an important lesson after my bout with postpartum thyroiditis. So, I acknowledged and reflected on the issue, had some testing done, and was surprised to find that I was dealing with not Stage 1 HPA axis dysfunction but Stage 3. If I'm honest with myself, the revealing conversation with my loved one probably needed to happen much sooner, and to this day, I still can't pinpoint when the whole stress problem started.

I share this story to illustrate a few things. First, if you can't tell, I can be a pretty stubborn person at times, particularly if it means admitting my own weaknesses. I love the illusion of self-sufficiency, and it requires a lot of humility for me to be able to recognize when I'm struggling. I want you to know that if you also find your health in disarray because of the stressors of motherhood, it doesn't mean there's something wrong with you. It doesn't mean you're a bad mom; it doesn't mean you aren't the precisely chosen, perfectly ordained parent for your baby; and it doesn't mean that you "just aren't cut out for this whole parenting thing." It also doesn't mean that you aren't a generally capable person. Rather, admitting your need for help—and getting it—paradoxically leads to less stress and the ability to live out this calling even more richly. But you first need to acknowledge your need for help.

Second, the stress that comes from parenting isn't as simple as thinking, "This requires work, and that work is hard for me to manage." Becoming a mother changes everything else about your life, especially relationships. Adding (another) baby to your life changes your family dynamic, in particular your relationship with your partner, as well as your relationship with your other children, if you have them. It completely overhauls your friendships, the way you relate to your own parents, your relationship to your work, and your relationship to God and your spiritual life. It's a wholly transformative transition that is truly unlike anything else we can experience on this side of heaven. For me, learning that I needed to rely on other people to successfully parent the way I needed to was, and is to this day, one of the hardest parts of motherhood. It has less to do with my babies and more with recognizing that I just can't do it all on my own. I need my husband and other family members in ways I didn't before. Such humility is hard, and it also forced me to confront a lot of really hard things in my past that led me to develop such a strong sense of self-reliance in the first place.

Maybe your stress, like mine, comes from recognizing that you can't—and were never meant to—do it all alone. Or maybe it comes from the fact that you don't have access to the help you need. Then there's the relational stress, the financial stress, the impact on your career, and all the other complexities that parenthood brings to our lives. Becoming a mother is amazing and transformative, but let's be honest—it's also stressful!

Please remember that stress comes in many forms and is not purely psychological. Physical stress also taxes the HPA system. This could be from sleeplessness itself—I have personally never been able to cope with sleep deprivation, as I end up on the verge of a panic attack until I can catch up. It could be from a calorie deficit or too much exercise too soon. It could be from physical pain or another physical disorder (like a thyroid condition or autoimmune disease) occurring alongside HPA axis dysfunction. Even exposure to pollution or chemicals in your environment can add to your body's overall stress load and throw off how your adrenal system works.

Finally, don't assume which stage you're in and self-treat. I shared earlier that, based on my symptoms, I'd guessed I was in Stage 1 of HPA axis dysfunction, but my test results demonstrated otherwise. Please note that HPA axis dysfunction (also known as adrenal dysfunction or general adaptation syndrome) reflects a disorder of the body's response to stress, brought on by chronic exposure to it. Additionally, keep in mind that this is not the only cause of dysfunctional cortisol output, as conditions like Addison's disease and Cushing's syndrome and malignancies like pheochromocytoma may also cause such symptoms. Accurate testing and a thorough medical workup in the diagnosis of HPA axis dysfunction or any other health problem are essential. Just like the symptoms of HPA axis dysfunction easily mimic normal postpartum symptoms, they also can just as easily mirror any of the other conditions outlined in this book and then some. I do not recommend self-diagnosing and attempting treatment for HPA axis dysfunction or any other condition explained in this book without first ensuring accurate diagnosis and collaborating with a healthcare provider, ideally one who is trained in the paradigm of functional medicine.

Treatment of HPA Axis Dysfunction

When it comes to actually treating HPA axis dysfunction, you need to first identify and name the source of your stress. Often, this is most easily and efficiently done with the help of a licensed mental healthcare provider, and it may even require medication like antianxiety drugs or antidepressants. Any stressor becomes even more difficult to cope with when a mental health condition is layered on top of it. Beyond medical management, however, counselors help build the organizational and coping skills required to live a full and vibrant life amid stressors. Some problems can't be fixed, and if a solution isn't immediately accessible, it doesn't mean you need to just suffer through it. Putting the appropriate supports in place or using the right tools at the right time can make all the difference.

Additionally, establishing healthy habits for sleep, nutrition, exercise, and other physical needs helps to keep your total stress load in check. Chapter 13 outlines these practices in detail, and truly, the strategies that I recommend my patients use to fix HPA axis dysfunction are the same things I recommend to anyone hoping to support their general sense of health and well-being. Pay special attention to nutrition, like getting enough food, eating enough protein, fiber, and fat to support healthy blood sugar levels, and avoiding excess sugar and carbohydrates. Refer to chapter 13 for details.

Finally, I also recommend the following strategies, specific to each stage of HPA axis dysfunction, to my patients as needed. Review them for yourself and bring them into conversation with your healthcare provider when putting together a treatment plan for adrenal dysfunction.

- *General Strategies for Adrenal Health*
  - In studies, omega-3 supplementation has been proven to prevent the adrenal activation caused by mental stress.[9] In addition to its cardiovascular and immune benefits, this is one more good reason to make sure you get enough omega-3s each day.
- *Stage 1 HPA Axis Dysfunction*
  - Vitamin C dosed at 1,000 mg helps maintain appropriate morning cortisol and dehydroepiandrosterone (DHEA) levels, particularly in groups with elevated cortisol levels first thing in the morning.[10]
  - Phosphatidylserine (400 mg) taken at times of elevated cortisol normalizes adrenal hyperresponsiveness following stress.[11]

- *Magnolia officinalis* (dosed at 500 mg/day of 1.5 percent standardized extract) has been shown in research to reduce cortisol levels in individuals with chronic stress.[12]

- *Stage 2 HPA Axis Dysfunction*
    - In studies, ashwagandha[13] and rhodiola taken at times of heightened stress, particularly morning and midday, decrease cortisol responses, improve energy, and increase mental performance. Clinical trials demonstrate effectiveness at 576 mg/day of rhodiola,[14] and dosage of ashwagandha varies. I usually start small with my patients, around 50–100 mg. Please note that too much ashwagandha can damage the liver, so it's important to use it under medical supervision.
- *Stage 3 HPA Axis Dysfunction*
    - Licorice root (the herb, not the candy) increases cortisol responsiveness in the body.[15] Please note that when used inappropriately, this effect of licorice can be damaging, so remember to consult a doctor first and only use under medical supervision.
    - In patients with chronically low cortisol output, such as Addison's disease, treatment with cortisol-mimicking drugs is essential. Adrenal glandular supplements, made from animal sources of adrenal cortex, contain active compounds with the same effect and can be used to support patients with low cortisol as seen in Stage 3 HPA axis dysfunction. Please remember that when used inappropriately this can be dangerous, so remember to consult a doctor first and only use under medical supervision.

- Salt intake increases cortisol levels,[16] a beneficial effect in individuals with low adrenal hormone output.[17] When clinically appropriate, I recommend that my patients with Stage 2 and 3 HPA axis dysfunction add a pinch of salt to each eight-ounce glass of water consumed.

CHAPTER 9

Insulin Resistance

How long does it take to lose the baby weight?"

According to Wordtracker.com, a database that documents the most common things that people type into search engines, this is the second most common query when it comes to postpartum body weight concerns.[1] It follows closely behind "How to lose the baby weight." In other words, postpartum women want to know how they can lose the weight they gained during pregnancy and how long it will take to do so. Here's my question: Is this something that *you* want to know?

In my experience, women typically ask these questions when they have already tried losing weight or are starting to wonder whether the amount of time it's taking them is normal. After all, the ones who seem to effortlessly bounce back after baby aren't likely spending precious time googling how to do something they've already done. Instead, it's those of us whose maternity clothes don't fit quite right anymore but who still can't pull on the prepregnancy jeans who start wondering if our experience is normal. Especially when paired with other new symptoms, like sugar cravings, insatiable hunger, and fatigue despite it all, we may start to wonder if our failed weight loss efforts reflect a deeper health condition. Based on my work with countless postpartum women describing such scenarios, it just might be so.

There is a wide range of what can be considered normal when it comes to postpartum weight loss. However, we do see evidence in scientific literature that achieving a pattern of weight loss by one year postpartum is very much the norm. A large cohort study published in 2020 found that 85 percent of women fell into a trajectory of steady postpartum weight loss within twelve months postpartum and achieved a pattern of weight maintenance by two years.[2] The 9.7 percent of women who did not lose weight at all and instead gained weight in the postpartum period were more likely to have gained more weight during pregnancy, with the postpartum result of worsened metabolic markers—such as higher fasting glucose and glycohemoglobin levels, higher cholesterol, and kidney and liver function markers—and increased inflammation by three years.[3] In other words, struggling to lose weight after childbirth is a red flag for a new mother's greater health status. So, what gives? It all comes down to the effects of insulin, an essential metabolic hormone, both during pregnancy and afterward.

The How and Why of Insulin and Body Fat

Jokes abound about "eating for two" during pregnancy, but I have yet to meet a pregnant mama who, upon seeing two pink lines on a First Response Early Result test, immediately starts serving herself double the portion she used to eat. Rather, most pregnant women I know seem to swing back and forth between nauseated aversions and insatiable cravings for culinary oddities, much to their own chagrin. Pregnancy weight gain, of course, involves more than just eating more food and gaining more body fat, considering that the baby, placenta, blood volume, and extra fluid all contribute meaningfully to the number on the scale increasing. The actual fat gains, on the other hand, depend largely on metabolic hormones that shift during pregnancy to favor body fat storage. Insulin in particular holds the responsibility for such growth of both mom and baby.

Insulin primarily helps healthy people control their blood sugar. Whenever we eat, our blood sugar increases and, in response, the pancreas secretes insulin to either help muscles use that sugar for energy or store the unused energy portion as body fat. During pregnancy, a metabolic shift occurs to favor increased blood sugar levels to support baby's growth as well as to promote body fat storage in mom to later use for breastfeeding. In situations where this process occurs in overdrive, gestational diabetes develops. While gestational diabetes reflects a loss of the body's ability to regulate this process, it happens a little bit in every pregnant woman—just like everyone should gain at least a little bit of body fat. As blood sugar and insulin levels rise during pregnancy, they are likewise also *supposed to* drop back down following delivery. Notice my emphasis on the phrase "supposed to." They should, but don't always. When they don't, insulin resistance or other metabolic disorders may develop.[4] Insulin resistance is to postpartum what gestational diabetes is to pregnancy: a metabolic disorder that makes it hard to regulate food intake, energy balance, inflammation, and growth.

While we primarily blame the placenta for such dysregulation of blood sugar and insulin levels during pregnancy, body fat cells themselves drive insulin resistance postpartum. We often think of body fat as simply a form of tissue that takes up space, but it does a lot more than that. Our fat cells are metabolically active, meaning that they create hormones, secrete cellular signaling molecules, and even release inflammatory products into the bloodstream, which then communicate with all other parts of the body. When fat cells grow, their metabolic activity dysregulates the production and utilization of insulin, causing insulin levels to rise. In the metabolic equation, more insulin means that the body therefore becomes preprogrammed to store food energy as body fat. While this is good and helpful during pregnancy, many postpartum women find it inconvenient when they'd prefer to lose weight. Worse, the condition of insulin resistance also brings symptoms of fatigue, pain, and skin changes, among others, which incidentally are often chalked up to just being part of the postpartum experience. Insulin resistance also may lead to recurrent yeast infections, increased thirst, or development of gout. Left unchecked, the metabolic effects of insulin resistance snowball over time, leading to potentially life-threatening chronic diseases like fatty liver disease, cardiovascular disease, type 2 diabetes, and more.

The Hallmark Symptom of Insulin Resistance

I screen all my patients for insulin resistance—pregnant, postpartum, or otherwise. This is because many people have no idea what insulin resistance is supposed to feel like, even if they've heard the term before. Though I wouldn't say that there's a good "textbook" definition for the symptoms shown by a patient with insulin resistance, I am much more likely to suspect this problem in my postpartum patients when the conversations circle around weight loss, or lack thereof, due to the statistical findings in the studies mentioned above. Like I mentioned before, most postpartum moms—roughly 85 percent of them—have firmly established a pattern of weight loss by the one-year mark.[5] Plus, as I've seen in my own patients, weight loss typically at least begins well before that. But when a new mom meets with me and laments that she weighs the exact same as she did—or maybe even more than—when she was forty weeks pregnant, my mental list of potential health concerns for her always includes the problem of insulin resistance.

Here's the thing, though: When my patients ask me about postpartum weight loss, I recognize that these questions are far from simple. They could represent anything from a woman needing direction for starting a weight loss program for the first time in her life to maybe a hidden cry for help from a new mom feeling lost, scared, and lonely amid a damaging relationship with food and a poor body image. They could be questions born from frustration that efforts that previously worked are no longer helpful, or perhaps expressions of worry that something else—like insulin resistance, hypothyroidism, or adrenal dysfunction—are hiding below the surface, wreaking havoc on a new mother's health. Often, my patients initiate these conversations with great courage because underwritten in them are deep-seated feelings of embarrassment and shame. What about you?

Regardless of the reason for your body weight concerns, there are a few main things that I always want to make sure my patients know and that I want to make sure that you know too:

1. You don't need to lose weight to be loved. Your weight loss or lack thereof is not a means for earning value, respect, or dignity. Your value and worth are inherent to your humanity. Neither losing nor gaining weight nor changing your body in any other way, shape, or form will change that.
2. You may not even need to lose weight for your health. Sometimes our desire for weight loss is purely cosmetic, and we may not realize this motivation in ourselves. This doesn't mean the desire is good or bad or holds any other moral value, but I want you to know that if your health is suffering, you can tangibly improve it even if the number on the scale doesn't change by a single ounce. On the other hand, if your body is healthy but you are unhappy with your weight, that's a different situation.
3. Body weight itself is not a disease. Changes to body fat levels or changes to how easily your body gains or loses weight may reflect a problematic shift in your biology, whether as part of a chronic disease or otherwise. These problems can be identified and addressed. However, it's not inherently problematic to look—or weigh—different postpartum than you did prepregnancy.
4. Even if you have insulin resistance, you still need to—and deserve to—eat. Please don't end up harming

> yourself in an attempt to help your health. If you feel lost in navigating your relationship to food and your body after giving birth, please reach out for help from a therapist or dietitian trained in postpartum health.

At the same time, I also understand that there are countless valid reasons for a woman to lose weight regardless of health implications. *That is okay.* You don't need to justify your desire for weight loss to anyone. This is not a book (or chapter) about weight loss, nor is it a book about body image. However, my heart for this chapter is for you to know that whether or not you are happy with your body weight has no bearing on whether or not your particular bodily changes—or lack thereof—reflect a metabolic disorder. More importantly, they in no way reflect your worth and value as a mother or as a human being deserving of dignity, respect, and love.

When Body Fat Signals a Problem

Changes to body fat levels or, in particular, difficulty losing weight postpartum may be a symptom of insulin resistance. The first way to start figuring out whether that's the case for you is to take a closer look at some of your other symptoms. Because insulin is a hormone that travels in the bloodstream to all other parts of the body, insulin resistance is likewise a whole-body metabolic disorder. Symptoms of it can and do show up in all parts of the body. Here are some of the most common symptoms that I see among postpartum moms that indicate the possibility of insulin resistance, in addition to weight gain and difficulty losing weight:

- **Aches and pains:** I mentioned earlier that insulin resistance is associated with inflammatory chemicals. Inflammation is responsible for the pain response, as well as redness and swelling. Sore, achy muscles and joints are common with insulin resistance because of this associated inflammation.[6]
- **Fatigue and brain fog:** With high insulin levels, the body favors energy storage over energy usage. This often comes at the expense of having enough energy for muscles to function freely. Likewise, the brain runs almost entirely on glucose![7] Not enough energy in the blood means not enough energy for brain and muscle activity.[8] Furthermore, inflammation notoriously makes you feel run down, fatigued, and foggy due to the immune processes involved.
- **Anxiety:** Fluctuations in blood sugar, particularly when blood glucose drops, commonly brings anxiety and even panic as a symptom.[9] Low blood sugar stresses the body, and that stress, for many, either triggers anxiety or physically feels like anxiety does (i.e., racing heart, insomnia, indigestion).
- **Depression:** Low energy often brings down everything else, like mood. Many people suffering with fatigue and physical discomfort fall into depression, which makes sense. It's hard to feel good-natured when you don't feel well, and insulin resistance is associated with higher rates of depression.[10]
- **Headaches:** Low blood sugar, high blood sugar, and insulin resistance–associated inflammation all may contribute to headaches, and insulin resistance

notoriously triggers migraines in those prone to them.[11]

- **Hot flashes:** Similar to the anxiety wrought by low blood sugar, insulin resistance often brings vasomotor symptoms, including hot flashes, sweating, or even night sweats.[12]
- **Acne:** High blood sugar levels, which often accompany insulin resistance, favor the growth of the inflammatory types of bacteria on the skin, which cause acne.[13] While postpartum hormone shifts commonly trigger acne, pimples that persist or develop after other expected postpartum symptoms fade away may signal a metabolic problem.

Testing for Insulin Resistance

Although insulin resistance is part of type 2 diabetes, they are not the same thing. Rather, insulin resistance reflects an earlier stage of metabolic dysfunction that could eventually develop into type 2 diabetes or a wide range of other chronic health conditions. Therefore, simply testing for whether or not someone's blood sugar levels reach high enough to warrant a type 2 diabetes diagnosis is not sufficient to identify insulin resistance. That being said, blood sugar testing does matter. Here's how I screen my patients for insulin resistance:

- **Fasting insulin:** One of the most accessible, accurate, and simplest methods for screening for insulin resistance is testing a person's blood levels of insulin while fasting, as insulin resistance means a person needs more insulin than usual to control their blood sugar.[14] But how high is too high? Research on groups of multiple thousands of individuals has demonstrated that those with normal glycemic responses and normal body mass index (BMI) have fasting insulin levels at or below 10 mIU/mL.[15] This is the reference range that I use when evaluating patient metabolic health in my practice. However, to screen specifically for insulin resistance, the research-informed cutoff is 16.3 mIU/mL.[16] Interestingly, both of these values are lower than the cutoff given by most laboratories.

- **Fasting glucose:** For most people, glucose levels should be low after a fasting period of eight to twelve hours, not high, as no food has been consumed. In individuals who struggle to control and lower blood sugar after meals, glucose levels may remain elevated for several hours after eating. While this does not screen for insulin resistance directly, it is widely accepted that a fasting blood sugar level above 110 mg/dL reflects increased odds of insulin resistance.[17] Please note that acute stress also elevates glucose levels—fasting or otherwise.[18] Elevations in this value followed by subsequent normal test results may reflect adrenal dysfunction.
- **Glycohemoglobin(A1c):** This red blood cell marker represents the average glucose level over the course of the RBC's lifespan, which is about three months. Whereas fasting glucose is a snapshot in time of blood sugar levels, A1c provides important historical context. An elevated A1c indicates chronic elevations in blood

sugar, a problem seen in insulin resistance as well as both prediabetes and type 2 diabetes. Individuals with A1c levels between 5.7 percent and 6.4 percent are widely accepted to be at increased risk of insulin resistance, though this test is not as specific or sensitive as other methods.[19]

A note about the oral glucose tolerance test (OGTT): The most widely accepted test for accurately diagnosing a problematic glycemic response is the OGTT, which is a test that was probably recommended to you at least once during pregnancy. Currently the standard for gestational diabetes screening, the OGTT involves drinking a sugar solution and completing a series of glucose blood tests at hour-long intervals thereafter. However, I do not routinely use this test in my practice because it's quite invasive, and most people feel ill after drinking that much sugar on an empty stomach—not to mention that doing so is far from healthy! Despite the accuracy of this testing method, plenty of other, less invasive and simpler screens exist, which are listed above, and which I recommend in lieu of the OGTT when screening for insulin resistance postpartum.

Treatment for Insulin Resistance

Currently, the number one recommended treatment for insulin resistance, according to the Endocrine Society's clinical practice guidelines, is lifestyle modification, primarily through exercise and dietary strategies that help support blood sugar control.[20] I agree completely with this strategy, and you can find additional recommendations for supporting a healthy glycemic response in chapter 13. However, both the Endocrine Society and I acknowledge that sometimes lifestyle modification is not enough. In these instances, doctors may prescribe the following:

- **Metformin:** This drug, which decreases absorption of carbohydrates from food and blocks liver activity, is usually the first-line treatment for disorders of glucose metabolism.
- **Thiazolidinediones, alpha-glucosidase inhibitors, orlistat:** These medications, among others, may also be prescribed, though they are not typically recommended due to the risk of adverse side effects.[21]

What about Glucagon-Like-Peptide-1 Agonist Drugs?

At the time that I am writing this book, GLP-1 agonists are not officially recommended for treatment of insulin resistance. However, these drugs are currently having a heyday for the purpose of weight loss. Given that as of 2022, nearly 45 percent of overweight young adults (age 18–44) were found to have insulin resistance,[22] it could be said that these GLP-1s are indeed prescribed routinely to insulin-resistant persons, mediating weight loss through the pathway of insulin sensitivity and metabolism. However, they are not recommended to be used while breastfeeding, which makes them a poor choice for postpartum women. They also are not recommended for women who are planning to become pregnant again in the imminent future.

In my practice, I also regularly offer the following therapies to be used in conjunction with diet and lifestyle strategies to support insulin regulation and metabolism:

- **Fenugreek:** This supplement has been well-demonstrated in clinical research to improve blood sugar control through mechanisms similar to metformin and GLP-1 agonist drugs.[23] Fenugreek also is effective at improving milk supply, making it a very appropriate herbal medicine for postpartum mothers with insulin resistance.[24]

- **Probiotics, vitamin D, vitamin C, zinc, and magnesium:** These supplements have also all been well-established in research to improve glucose control and insulin resistance.[25] Many of these have been covered in previous chapters, so I won't repeat the details here. They also are all considered safe for use while breastfeeding. Please note that not all probiotics are created equal, but those containing several different strains of bacteria at high doses have the best evidence for improving insulin resistance.[26] Look for ingredient labels that have fifty billion or more colony-forming units (CFU) and more than one type of listed microbe (e.g., *Lactobacillus rhamnosus*, *Bifidobacterium longum*, *Saccharomyces boulardii*).
- **Berberine:** This herb has comparable efficacy to metformin in clinical trials, regulates the insulin response, and reduces inflammation.[27] Please note that this should not be used long-term due to possible adverse effects on the gut microbiome. I do not routinely recommend berberine to breastfeeding women or for periods longer than three months.

CHAPTER 10

Pelvic Floor Dysfunction

I tried not to laugh as my best friend modeled transversus abdominis breathing to me on her living room floor, a look of almost pained concentration on her face. Twenty-one years old, fresh out of college, and excited to take the next steps of my medical career, I thought I knew it all. But I'd never even heard of diastasis recti, and yet there, right in front of me, was a living, breathing, exercising model. After giving birth, my friend shared with me that her abdominal muscles had separated from each other, and she was paying thousands of dollars out of pocket for a specialized form of physical therapy to correct it.

"Why doesn't insurance cover it?" I asked her, astounded at the four-figure sum she'd be paying to complete her treatment.

"They clearly don't believe that this is a real problem," she groaned, trying to talk while coordinating contractions from muscles she hadn't used correctly for nine months. As she did so, I saw a strip of tissue pushing outward from a three-inch-wide ridge on her abdomen, stretching from the center of her rib cage to her belly button. It looked like a large skin-colored hot dog was poking out of her belly and then receding back into it.

"Well, then they need to take a look at your abs—then they'll see that it is!" I replied. We devolved into laughter, and my friend gave up on her exercise session for the day. I went home and filed away the information I'd learned during my visit:

1. Pelvic floor dysfunction is a thing.
2. Many doctors and insurance companies aren't aware of it.
3. I should be on the lookout for it in the future, whether for myself or others.

Fast-forward a few years to my internship. I was working at a multidisciplinary clinic that also had acupuncturists and physical therapists on staff. During my first-day tour, I learned that one of the PTs specialized in—of all things—pelvic floor physical therapy. Recalling my friend's experience with diastasis recti, I asked her if I could shadow her on one of my days off, and she graciously agreed. After receiving consent from each patient for me to be in the room, I watched her evaluate the muscular tone, contractility, symmetry, and strength of each patient's abdomen, hips, and pelvic floor, including both an external and an internal examination. It was the most comprehensive pelvic exam I'd ever seen, far more detailed than even the palpations performed at well-woman exams. The physical therapist narrated to me each body part that she evaluated, naming small muscles that I hardly remembered, as three years had passed since I'd completed my anatomy courses: "Obturator internus 4/5, iliococcygeus 3/5, ischiococcygeus 3/5 . . ."

During our lunch break that day, the physical therapist explained that, like me, she also had never learned anything about pelvic floor physical therapy in her graduate program, apart from the fact that it exists. "I had to complete a course consisting of two thousand hours of specialized training *after* graduation to get certified to perform pelvic rehabilitation. It's a very niche area," she noted, "and I've had to educate a lot of referring providers myself. Many doctors just don't know about it, and patients don't, either, until I tell them, of course. But it's a really common problem among women."

I thought back to a patient encounter from that morning, when the woman graciously explained to me that she'd initially been referred to the clinic because of back pain. She was shocked to learn that the problem was not her back, in fact, but her pelvic floor.

"I've been in PT so many times before, and I'd get better for a little while, but it just kept coming back," she lamented. "So even though I was a little skeptical about this pelvic floor stuff, I was willing to try just about anything to fix the problem. I even had doctors recommend surgery to me! Can you imagine"—she looked me in the eye—"I might have had spinal surgery, when the issue was—*this*—a completely separate part of my body." I nodded in understanding and thanked her for sharing her experience with me. When I went home that evening, I again filed away what I'd learned:

1. Even most physical therapists have no idea what pelvic floor physical therapy entails.

2. Misdiagnosis among postpartum women is a huge, huge issue, even in the musculoskeletal world.
3. Herman & Wallace is the name of the educational institution where pelvic floor PTs receive their training. Patients can search via the tool on their website to find certified providers.

Fast-forward another few years to where I was standing in my sister's kitchen at a family party, seven months pregnant with my first baby. I was talking to my aunt when I sneezed. "Oh my gosh!" I whispered, and I ran to the bathroom to see if my suspicions were true. Indeed, they were—I had leaked some urine due to the force of the sneeze plus the several-pounds-and-growing baby sitting on my bladder. However, this wasn't the first time that had happened. I'd actually already been wearing a pad for precisely that reason.

After getting changed, I returned to the kitchen and apologized to my aunt with the hope of nonchalantly resuming conversation. She smiled knowingly and patted me on the shoulder. "Welcome to the club, honey," she said. "It only gets worse with menopause." Bemused, I once again filed away the information I'd learned that day:

1. *Stress incontinence*, the technical term for leaking urine with sudden, increased abdominal pressure, is so common among women of all ages that it's almost a rite of passage.
2. Many women take for granted that pelvic floor dysfunction is just part of life and don't realize that it can be helped.

3. The muscle loss of menopause exacerbates pelvic weakness wrought by pregnancy, causing the problem to worsen with age if early intervention isn't available.

Another year passed, and I was in my office at my desk, with Betty sitting across from me. She explained that she was going to be having surgery and wanted to know which supplements and medications, if any, she needed to stop before going under anesthesia. I was a little taken aback, as I'd been meeting with Betty roughly every month since we started treatment for her acne, and she'd never mentioned this surgery to me. She was a marathon runner with no pain, no historical injury, no illness that I was aware of, and I suddenly worried that I'd missed something important about her health history. I quickly scanned my notes to see if I could catch my mistake and then finally asked, "I'm sorry, remind me which surgery you'll be having?"

"Oh, um . . ." Her eyes dropped to the floor. "I guess I didn't mention it to you. I'm going to be having a bladder sling procedure." I cocked my head slightly, waiting for her to finish. "It's so embarrassing," she started, and tears suddenly started to fill her eyes, but she choked them back and continued. "With my long runs in particular, when I get tired, the leakage is just so much. It's more than I can control anymore. So, after the marathon this weekend, I'm going to have the surgery. I've already met with a urologist, and he thinks I'm a good candidate for it. It's scheduled for next week."

My heart sank a bit further with each word. In the back of my mind, I heard the echoes of previous conversations that I'd filed away for precisely a moment such as this. I saw my best friend laughing while she tried to demonstrate pelvic tilts to me on her living room floor the summer after I graduated from college. I heard the patient at the multidisciplinary clinic explaining how desperate she was for relief. I saw my aunt's cheeky grin as she welcomed me into the urinary incontinence club. But I mostly saw myself walking into my own first appointment for pelvic floor physical therapy, just a few months prior, to start my own process of healing my pelvic floor after childbirth, feeling nervous but hopeful.

"Betty, I totally understand," I started. "Thank you for telling me about the surgery. It's important for me to know about that aspect of your health. I'm sorry I didn't ask about that symptom earlier." She raised an eyebrow at me, and I continued to explain how I'd just graduated from my own three-month-long pelvic floor treatment program and how much it had helped my own symptoms of urinary leakage when laughing, coughing, sneezing, or jumping. "Let's be honest, though," I joked, "I still don't plan on using a trampoline any time soon, just to be safe . . ."

Betty noted that her doctor never even mentioned that physical therapy was an option, and like so many other women, she'd had no idea. We talked through the details of how it works and what it involves and shared our frustrations that this area of women's health had been neglected for so long.

"I wish I knew about this sooner," she said, "because I might have made a different decision." She explained that she was still going to have the surgery but was grateful for what I'd shared. However, this had been such a heart-wrenching and difficult decision for her to make, and even though she was scared, she was at peace with it. "I already have a plan, and even if my recovery takes longer than expected, I should still have enough wiggle room to start training for the Chicago Marathon next fall."

And that's exactly what she did. Betty underwent the bladder sling surgery with great success, recovered well, and was able to return to her training schedule right on time. I was happy for Betty, but sad at the same time, both for her and for all the other women who underwent invasive, painful surgeries without full awareness of all of their options. I wondered, on Betty's behalf, what could have been. Would pelvic floor PT have worked for her? What about the strength of her other pelvic muscles? Would she return to running marathons on a weak obturator internus, basically becoming a ticking time bomb for a hip injury? Obviously, there is no right or wrong answer when it comes to these sorts of healthcare decisions, but I know that many women would prefer to avoid surgery and prevent future injury, given the choice. I know I would.

Inspired to change as much as I could for as many women as possible, I made a new practice of asking specifically about the symptom of urinary incontinence at every new patient examination. Ironically, to this day, the only provider who has ever asked *me* about this symptom was my own pelvic floor physical therapist, whom I was seeing specifically for the purpose of treating it. Be the change you wish to see in the world.

The Pelvic Floor and All Its Associated Problems

We already explored in chapter 2 how the pelvis and its associated muscles shift during pregnancy, creating weakness in some areas as well as tightness and even pain in others. These muscle imbalances lead to debilitating and often embarrassing symptoms for women after they deliver their babies. While in the first few weeks postpartum we expect soreness, changes in sensation, and other transient abnormalities, persistent pain, urinary leakage, constipation, prolapse, and recurrent urinary tract infections are never normal—no matter how common they might be. Pelvic floor dysfunction can bring about all these problems and more. Here's an overview of some of the more common pelvic floor–associated problems I see in my practice and why they develop postpartum:

- **Diastasis recti (DR):** Caused by abdominal expansion during pregnancy, the abdominal muscles separate and sometimes remain so postpartum. This leads to outpouching of abdominal organs and tissue. In addition to creating pelvic instability and susceptibility to injury, DR creates the appearance of an abdominal "pooch," which many women mistake for belly fat. Ironically, continuing to exercise without strengthening the necessary muscles reinforces dysfunctional movement patterns that can make the problem worse. DR produces a characteristic sausage-like bulge or "doming" appearance of the belly with abdominal contraction.
- **Painful sex, vaginismus, vulvodynia, and other pelvic pain:** Weak muscles that fail to contract correctly as well as short, tight, and inflamed muscles can lead to spasming, cramping, and generalized pelvic pain. This is exacerbated for many women during sex, while using tampons, during bowel movements, or during some types of exercise. Because the pelvic muscles stretch due to hormonal shifts and the physical weight

of pregnancy, these pain syndromes affect both women who delivered their babies vaginally as well as those who undergo C-section.

- **Pelvic organ prolapse:** Due to the weakening of ligaments and muscles of the pelvis, organs like the uterus, cervix, bowel, and bladder sometimes protrude through the muscular walls of the vagina, creating sensations of pressure, fullness, or pain. Sometimes the bulging is visible in the external vulvar area. Prolapse may lead to urinary retention, increasing risk of urinary tract infections and kidney infections.
- **Incontinence:** Leakage of urine or stool due to weakness of the muscles designed to hold waste creates embarrassment, shame, and tremendous inconvenience for many women.
- **Inability to achieve orgasm:** Uncoordinated pelvic muscle contraction or weak muscles may affect the level of function necessary for sexual pleasure or orgasm.
- **Recurrent urinary tract infections:** Poor tone of pelvic muscles may obstruct the urethra or bladder, trapping urine, which harbors bacteria.
- **Urinary frequency and urgency:** Whether or not incontinence is present, muscular imbalances may lead to increased urinary pressure or strong urges to use the bathroom despite passing small amounts of urine. This affects sleep as well as quality of life.
- **Constipation and hemorrhoids:** Weakness and tightness of the pelvic muscles both can lead to difficulty passing stool. Many women report the urge to go but

find it difficult to find the right position to allow the stool to pass. Unintended withholding of stool can lead to tension of the rectal veins, possibly producing hemorrhoids, as well as hard, dry stools, bloating, cramping, and even nausea or heartburn.

- **Pain in hips, buttocks, low back, and legs:** The nerves that allow muscle contraction and provide sensation to the hips and legs originate in the spinal cord and stretch down through the pelvis. Tightness of the pelvic muscles or prolapse of pelvic organs can "pinch" nerves, leading to sharp, shooting pains and other changes to sensation or muscle strength. Weakness of the abdominal and pelvic muscles also creates instability in the back, core, and lower extremities, predisposing postpartum women to injuring themselves through even seemingly basic movements.

Treatment for Pelvic Floor Dysfunction

Fixing the problem of imbalanced muscles in the pelvic floor starts with a pelvic floor exam. This includes evaluation of the pelvic floor muscles (muscles stretching from the pubic bone to the tail bone) as well as the muscles that support and provide stability to the pelvis (including glutes, hamstrings, abdominal muscles, and back muscles). During the initial exam, a pelvic floor physical therapist will evaluate the strength, flexibility, tension, and symmetry of each of these muscles. Examination involves both internal (akin to gynecological exams) and external (i.e., "Hold your leg up and don't let me push it down") components. You'll be asked to change into a gown and, particularly if you are experiencing pain as a symptom, you might feel a little nervous when the appointment starts. However, pelvic floor PTs are trained to be respectful, communicative, and gentle, so the exam shouldn't hurt.

A note about pelvic floor examination in physical therapy: Internal exams are a little uncomfortable for everyone but particularly for women who have experienced physical or sexual abuse, a traumatic delivery, miscarriage, or stillbirth. In these cases, they may be outright unbearable. If this describes you, there are a few things I want you to know. First, I'm so sorry this has been your experience, but I assure you that there is hope for healing. You are not alone. Second, if you haven't already, please make an appointment with a licensed mental health professional with experience in your area of trauma. Healing happens in community, and your healthcare team is part of that. It is our privilege and honor to help you in this journey. And finally, please know that pelvic floor physical therapy doesn't need to happen right now if you're not ready. It's okay to wait, work through other aspects of your health first, and circle back when it's the right time.

Once the pelvic floor therapist has made a diagnosis, they will prescribe a treatment plan that involves anything from breathing techniques and manual therapy (massage, trigger point release) to stretching and targeted exercises designed to restore strength and stability to all the muscles of the pelvis, core, and extremities. Some physical therapy offices even offer biofeedback technology, acupuncture or dry needling, electrical stimulation, cryotherapy, ultrasound, thermography, and magnetic stimulation. Your treatment plan is also guaranteed to include at-home exercises. Please hear me when I say that consistency with the at-home program is essential. Rehab exercises don't work unless you do them!

Depending on the individual muscles involved in your condition and the treatment modalities available at your clinic, your treatment plan should be unique and tailored specifically to you. That being said, here are a few broad lifestyle habits and strategies for the purpose of supporting pelvic health that apply to everyone postpartum:

- **Rest, rest, rest:** It probably goes without saying that giving birth is like running a marathon. It's normal to feel bruised and sore postpartum, and you should use these bodily cues as a reminder to stay put. Give your body the chance to recover, because if you don't, you will increase your risk of injuring yourself and creating bigger problems with your pelvic health.
- **Stretch:** Imagine lifting a bag of groceries from the floor. Doing so requires a decent amount of strength, especially if there are a few gallons of milk in the bag. Now, imagine lifting that same bag of groceries, but instead of starting from the floor, you lift them up off a stool that's waist-height. It would be easier, right? Long muscles are strong because there's a greater length or distance to perform the work of muscular contraction. On the flip side, short and tight muscles tend to be weak (because there's less distance required to complete the movement). As you receive the all clear to get back into exercise postpartum, make sure you stretch first! I understand that doing so requires time, and that time—especially when pieced together between naps—is so very precious. But in addition to allowing greater strength and stability, stretching prevents injury.

- **Use a bathroom stool:** If you haven't yet invested in a Squatty Potty (or a knockoff version of one), now is the time to do so. Tight pelvic floor muscles make it difficult for stool to pass through, and you can strain your pelvic floor by pushing. Instead, elevating your feet off the floor to bend your knees during bowel movements forces the pelvic floor to relax and allows for smoother, gentler, and safer movements. It is also worth mentioning that we should avoid spending too much time sitting on the toilet, as this also can strain the pelvic floor. If a bowel movement doesn't happen within a few minutes, take a break and try again later when the urge returns.
- **Pay attention to your posture:** In addition to bathroom posture, take note of how you sit and stand. In general, when standing, your knees, hips, and shoulders should all be in line with each other. Jutting your hip forward or hiking your weight onto one hip allows your core to get lazy, and your core strength is an essential player in your pelvic stability. Likewise, try to avoid slumping in chairs. If you notice yourself doing it, prop yourself up on pillows to relax into the correct posture.
- **Breathe in, breathe out:** Using the correct muscles for breathing is another essential piece of core stability and pelvic health. In my experience, many of us do it wrong, possibly because we've been programmed by our culture to "suck it in" as much as possible. Allow your breath—and yourself—to take up space. When inhaling, think about relaxing your whole body,

especially your belly, to allow it to naturally expand. When exhaling, imagine that you're zipping up your abdomen from your pubic bone up to your ribs. A pelvic floor PT can help make sure you're breathing correctly, as it can be really tricky to identify the correct muscles. However, these visuals can be a helpful starting point while you await your first appointment.

Before closing, I wanted to share one last note about insurance coverage. Although we are still worlds behind where we should be in the field of women's health, we have come a long way since that early conversation with my friend who paid out of pocket for her pelvic floor treatment. In my experience of referring patients to pelvic floor physical therapy, more and more insurance companies in the US are willing to pay for pelvic floor PT, just like any other condition. Moreover, because this treatment niche is increasing in popularity among physical therapy providers, cash programs are becoming more accessible. I personally was able to find a pelvic floor physical therapist affiliated with the women's health department at a local hospital, and my health insurance covered my visits in full. I often refer my patients either to hospitals or to an affordable subscription-based program I've found near Chicago. I also truly believe that when it comes to your health, the right provider is worth investing in. If you need help finding a pelvic-trained PT, check out the "Find a Practitioner" tool at HermanWallace.com.

Note: Pelvic floor physical therapy can help alleviate the pain associated with endometriosis, interstitial cystitis (a painful bladder condition), as well as any of the other problems listed earlier, even if they weren't found to be caused by pregnancy and childbirth. If you experience pain, instability, or any other form of discomfort in your low back, pelvis, hips, or lower extremity, consider making an appointment with a pelvic floor physical therapist (or asking your doctor for a referral if you live in a state that requires one). Pelvic floor physical therapists are trained in evaluating the whole body, just like any other physical therapist. They simply bring extra tools for diagnosis and treatment to the table when evaluating conditions of the female body.

CHAPTER 11

Depression, Anxiety, and Other Mental Health Concerns

We have now arrived at possibly the most important and yet the most controversial of all topics in the postpartum sphere, as it speaks to the quality-of-life experiences of motherhood. Despite being one of the most well-known postpartum conditions and the *only one* thus far for which the American College of Obstetrics and Gynecology recommends routine screening, half of postpartum depression (PPD) cases still go undiagnosed.[1] As with all the other conditions we've already discussed, you can't get help for postpartum depression, or any other health problem, if you never knew you were dealing with it in the first place.

Thanks to increased awareness of PPD and the routine screenings administered in both gynecology and pediatric offices, most of us have heard of postpartum depression. Given that it affects more than 13 percent of postpartum women, you probably personally know someone who has struggled with it.[2] Moreover, most of us already understand the risks of undiagnosed and untreated cases, ranging from loss of joy and missed opportunities to relationship problems, attachment problems, and the worst-case scenario (which is, for many of us, among our greatest fears): death. In this chapter, the most pressing question is not about what postpartum depression is but how and why we so often mistake it for just a normal part of the postpartum experience.

One of the biggest reasons for underdiagnosis among PPD patients is the fact that women don't recognize the symptoms in themselves and therefore don't realize that the idea of getting help is even relevant. All kinds of research endeavors show results like this, with one 2014 study finding that an alarming 40 percent of women with symptoms of PPD never seek help for it.[3] But it's not because we're oblivious to the fact of our hardships; it's because motherhood is so inherently challenging and overhauls our lifestyles so dramatically that we struggle to identify the line between "normal hard" and a mental health issue. Take my friend Jessica, for example, whom I shared about in chapter 4. She altogether didn't realize that she was experiencing depression and even thought she was doing pretty well (all things considered) until *after* her mental health got better. The hindsight provided clarity she just didn't have while in the thick of it.

For me personally, feelings of depression were absolutely a part of my thyroid condition. It was hard not to get down in the dumps when I couldn't get off the couch and simple things, such as getting food for myself, took every ounce of energy I could muster. I was unmotivated and disengaged, and everything was covered in a generalized sense of fogginess—like I couldn't think in color. Both Jessica and I thought our experiences were normal, and I in particular spent a lot of time trying to convince myself of this despite some suspicions to the contrary. Truthfully, motherhood *is* hard, and often it's a struggle to know where our babies end and we begin—much less to gather the self-awareness needed to realize that we might be dealing with a diagnosable (and treatable) mental health issue.

Note: Depression and anxiety during the postpartum period are diagnosed as such when there isn't another explanation for why the symptoms are occurring. That being said, anything from nutrient deficiencies to thyroid disease and adrenal problems can show up with depression or anxiety as symptoms, which resolve when the root cause is addressed. Please take caution not to view these mental health symptoms as a totally separate issue from your physical health; they can be and often are a symptom of a larger postpartum health problem, which is why a thorough screening and workup are essential. Healing your mental health often also requires identifying and healing other dysfunctions in your physical body.

Then there's the fact that postpartum mental health involves much more than depression. There's postpartum anxiety (PPA), postpartum obsessive-compulsive disorder (OCD), postpartum post-traumatic stress disorder (PTSD), and even the rare but extremely serious postpartum psychosis. We might say to ourselves, "I'm not depressed. I'm happier than I've ever been," despite feeling "off" in some way or experiencing concerning symptoms. These other conditions don't share the same notoriety as PPD, so it's easier for a mom struggling with debilitating anxiety to set her mental health aside because she doesn't realize that she might be dealing with a condition related to her postpartum state. "I've always been anxious," she might say. "I didn't have time to address it before the baby came, and now I certainly don't." What about you? Did you know that there's a special kind of anxiety with its very own name that affects postpartum moms? How about postpartum OCD? Or PTSD?

Even outside of these diagnosable conditions, numerous other *normal* postpartum mental health experiences exist, muddying the water, and themselves sometimes bring guilt and shame that get in the way of seeking help. These include things like the baby blues and intrusive thoughts, which many providers never educate pregnant mothers about. Then, when they occur, they can be so alarming that a new mom doesn't know how to wrap her mind around them, much less how to take the next step. And now we see why half of postpartum women struggle to identify a mental health issue and seek treatment for it! It's all just so complicated.

Postpartum mental health is such a sensitive and complex subject that I don't have enough space in this chapter to cover everything that needs to be said or explained. Thankfully, there are countless books on these subjects, and if you suspect, even for a moment, that you are dealing with a mental health concern, please reach out to any member of your healthcare team. Whether that be the provider who helped you deliver your baby, a primary care doctor, a provider at an urgent care clinic, a therapist or mental health counselor, or a provider in any other health discipline, any and all of them can connect you with local, accessible referrals to get help. If you are so overwhelmed that you have no idea where to start, begin with the

National Maternal Mental Health Hotline (available in both English and Spanish): 1-833-852-6262.

Now, as for this chapter, here's what we do have the space to cover: the symptoms of postpartum depression and postpartum anxiety (the two most common postpartum mental health conditions), at what point those symptoms signify a transition from normal to pathological, and what your options are for addressing them. I also want to make very, very clear the following:

1. Postpartum mental health conditions are extremely common. While they are not normal, and you deserve help and support in managing them, you are not alone in your struggles.
2. Mental health struggles are not your fault. Just like autoimmunity, thyroid conditions, or nutrient deficiencies, they reflect the fact that we live in a broken world in which many things are not as they should be.
3. You are not a bad mom. Feeling overwhelmed by your postpartum journey, whether it be your first baby or your fifth, in no way reflects your fitness for the job, the quality of your parenting, your love for any of your children, or anything else about who you are.
4. Today's struggle will not last forever. Even though you are and will be forever changed by the experience of motherhood, mental health evolves over time. You may need support for a little while, but that doesn't mean you will forever. Seeing a therapist, starting a medication, or even just admitting and naming your struggle is not a lifelong diagnosis.

What Is and Isn't Normal with Maternal Mental Health

Did your doctor talk to you about the baby blues? If not, I will right now.

In my conversations with postpartum women, I've noticed a lot of confusion between the baby blues and postpartum depression, with these two terms often used interchangeably. The truth is, the baby blues are a normal experience of emotional instability, including weepiness, irritability, and anxiety, and may also include difficulty sleeping, lack of motivation, feelings of overwhelm or exhaustion, difficulty concentrating, and changes in appetite. Affecting up to 80 percent of postpartum women,[4] the baby blues start within a few days of giving birth, and most sources state that they should resolve within two to three weeks postpartum.

The symptoms of the baby blues are just about the same as the symptoms of postpartum depression or anxiety, though the key difference is the time frame. Whereas the baby blues start soon after giving birth and resolve within a few weeks, postpartum depression can start any time within the first year after delivery.[5] While postpartum anxiety doesn't officially carry the same one-year time frame for diagnosis, both conditions can develop soon after delivery, or they may wait to begin for the first time after several months. The notable red flag is that the symptoms last longer than two weeks and that the feelings they bring begin to affect our behavior. We'll touch on more of what this looks like in a bit.

The other area of perinatal mental health that warrants discussion as we differentiate normal from not normal is the problem of intrusive thoughts. Intrusive thoughts are sudden, unwanted, and often upsetting or profoundly distressing thoughts or mental images that pop up and sometimes feel difficult to control. Many times these thoughts center around the health and safety of our children, our other family members, or ourselves, but they really can be about anything. A common intrusive thought, in my experience talking with both patients and other providers in the mental health field, centers around babies and stairs or heights. For example, a new mom may suddenly have a flashing mental image of a baby falling down the stairs or over a railing. Such a thought might occur at a completely random time, unrelated to actually using the stairs, or even in a mom whose home doesn't have any stairs!

Intrusive thoughts of this nature are distressing enough to begin with, considering the horror of something bad happening to our precious, vulnerable new little babies. But sometimes the most terrifying part of them is that they bring thoughts of intentional harm. Intrusive thoughts may therefore include: (1) thoughts of accidental harm (i.e., "What if I tripped and fell down the stairs while holding my baby?"), as well as (2) thoughts of intentional harm (i.e., "What if I walked up to the stair railing and dropped my baby over it?") Shocking and scary as both these thoughts are, what may surprise you even more is that both of them are *normal.* A 2024 study published in the *Journal of Clinical Psychiatry* found that 95.8 percent of postpartum women experience unwanted thoughts of accidental harm, and 53.9 percent experience unwanted thoughts of intentional harm.[6]

Not only do nearly all women experience intrusive thoughts of some type in the postpartum period, it's important to remember that under normal circumstances, they are *unwanted.* They are distressing, repulsive, and scary. They don't make sense, and we recognize that they are untrue. This is important in differentiating from other forms of more severe psychiatric illnesses, such as postpartum psychosis, in which the intrusive thoughts don't seem outlandish or abnormal to the affected mother. To differentiate further, intrusive thoughts are normal when they repulse us. They become red flags when they seem appealing or bring feelings of relief when they occur to us. In both cases, it's still a good idea to seek help, because the distress caused by even normal intrusive thoughts is, well, distressing. Trained mental health providers like counselors and therapists can equip you with cognitive techniques to cope with the intrusive thoughts, help them to become less frequent, and recover from them more quickly when they occur.

That brings me to the next piece of our discussion about distressing thoughts, anxiety, or depressive symptoms and the point at which they begin to affect behavior. Here's an example from my own life: Since becoming a mother, I have often struggled with intrusive thoughts surrounding the safety and well-being of my children. One such fear relates to train tracks and what would happen if my car stalled while I was driving over them. I could not, for the life of me, tell you how this fear originated. I think my brain just invented it one day, but I'd never even thought about it until after having children. Images of horrific train-related scenarios pop into my head every few months in totally unrelated circumstances, and sometimes even when I'm sleeping. I wake up drenched in sweat, my heart pounding, absolutely sure the next railroad crossing I drive through will be the end of me and my whole family. The only way I'm able to fall back asleep is by repeating to myself over and over again that my children are safely sleeping in their beds, which are nowhere near any train tracks. For the most part, outside of these troubling moments, I carry on with my life without much train-related worry.

However, if out of this fear I develop the habit of avoiding driving over train tracks, or perhaps avoiding driving at all, then I would have a problem. Intrusive thoughts are normal, but changing our behavior in response to them is not. Likewise, modifying my behavior because of anxiety would be a red flag for needing help because the anxiety would then be affecting my ability to live my life normally. The same is true with depressive symptoms—if I were to feel so exhausted, low in motivation, or down in the dumps that I neglected to do important tasks of daily life, like taking a shower or bringing my children to the doctor, it would be a sign of a significant problem in need of help. Anxious or depressive symptoms that caused me to lose my joy, affected my ability to think clearly, or got in the way of me doing things I otherwise once enjoyed would be a sign that I was dealing with something more than mere overwhelm and more than "just adjusting to parenthood." Those symptoms would have meant that I needed help.

I also want to point out that the baby blues of those early weeks postpartum also may cause some confusion for new moms because of the problem of relativity. Here's what I mean: If the baby blues were to continue at the same intensity for several months, it would be clear that the mom was dealing with a significant mental health crisis. However, the short-lived nature of these symptoms and their near ubiquity make them appear as a normal part of the postpartum experience rather than a pathology. Let's say, though, that after one to two weeks the intensity of the symptoms dies down and some of them resolve altogether. Perhaps for the first two weeks, a mom experiences trouble sleeping, feelings of overwhelm, plus complete exhaustion. She also finds herself feeling panicky for a few days because her life has changed so dramatically, and she wonders if she really was ready for this tiny baby with such big needs. But as the days pass, both mom and baby fall into a sleep rhythm, making life feel less overwhelming. Mom's energy levels improve a bit, and she is able to resume some of her previous activities, like taking walks, reading a few novels, and cooking. By the end of the first month, she's starting to feel like she's settling into parenthood, and she has a better idea of what her new normal will look like.

However, the anxiety lingers. The short fuse persists. She has far less tolerance for sensory stimulation. Although she's mostly sleeping when the baby sleeps, she can't nap despite her best efforts (and despite her tiredness) because of racing thoughts about her to-do list, worries about exposures during cold and flu season, and how she is going to find a way to fit pumping into her work schedule when her maternity leave ends. Every spare moment is spent researching rates of influenza in her area and worrying about whether to allow her in-laws to drop off a meal. *What if they forget to wash their hands?*

Maybe you don't share any of the same concerns as this hypothetical mother. However, what I want you to pay attention to is the fact that even if your symptoms improve after the first two weeks, improvement doesn't equal *resolution*. You still may be struggling with your mental health, but just because it's not as bad as it was at the beginning doesn't mean it isn't worth looking into at all. Meanwhile, simply exploring the idea of mental health support doesn't mean that you need to do any specific thing or anything at all about it. This is simply an invitation to make an honest assessment of how you're feeling and whether that, to you, is what you envision as thriving or not. If it's anything less, mama, you deserve better!

How to Get Help for Postpartum Depression and Anxiety

The number one most effective therapy for postpartum depression and anxiety is cognitive behavioral therapy (CBT), a psychotherapy technique that systematically helps patients reframe negative thoughts and, subsequently, negative behavior patterns.[7] In effect, recipients of CBT are able to create new ways of thinking, with improvements in mood, temperament, and cognitive function. Other forms of talk therapy have also shown effectiveness in improving postpartum mood disorders.

In my experience, many psychiatric and even primary care providers also prescribe medication, especially selective serotonin reuptake inhibitors (SSRIs) like sertraline. However, there are a few things to note about use of SSRIs for treatment of postpartum mood disorders. The first is that there is no shame in using a medication for this or any other purpose. If it's needed, it's needed—and you deserve to think and feel in the healthiest ways possible. That being said, according to the research, use of SSRIs is not more effective than treatment with cognitive behavioral therapy,[8] which actually has been studied more extensively in treatment of postpartum mood disorders than medication. Furthermore, when considering the root cause, lack of social support is the most modifiable risk factor for developing postpartum depression.[9] Psychotherapy directly addresses that need. For this reason, I recommend psychotherapy not only to patients exhibiting signs and symptoms of postpartum depression or anxiety but to all postpartum moms. I find it tremendously helpful as an additional source of social support in our highly individualistic and increasingly isolated culture.

In the realm of functional medicine, we also know of additional, breastfeeding-safe tools for improving mental health in the postpartum period, particularly regarding anxiety and depression. These include:

- **Exercise:** Approximately eighty minutes per week of moderate intensity exercise like walking, which most women can safely complete soon after delivery, as well as cycling and resistance training reduce risk of postpartum depression and anxiety by 45 percent.[10]
- **Omega-3 fatty acids:** Omega-3 fatty acid supplements with a high ratio of EPA/DHA demonstrated significant efficacy in treatment of both mild-to-moderate perinatal and postpartum depression with minimized risk of side effects.[11] Refer back to chapter 5 regarding nutrient deficiencies for information regarding safe supplementation with omega-3s.
- **Vitamin D:** Although the mechanism is not as well understood as other types of depression, systematic review studies identified a direct relationship between vitamin D status and perinatal mental health. Risk of PPD was found to be greatest among women with the lowest vitamin D levels.[12] Refer back to chapter 5 for more details on supplementation.
- **Curcumin:** Randomized controlled trials demonstrate that 500 mg per day of curcumin decreases perinatal depression and anxiety scores.[13]

Edinburgh Postnatal Depression Scale (EPDS)

The following questionnaire is a research-validated tool for postpartum depression screening, currently regarded as the standard of care for screening in obstetric offices. It was developed by J. L. Cox, J. M. Holden, and R. Sagovsky and published in the *British Journal of Psychiatry* in 1987.[1]

To complete the questionnaire, answer each question to the best of your ability. The point score for each answer is located in parentheses at the end of each response option. If you score 1–3 points on question 10, or the sum of points for all questions is greater than 11, or if you have any concerns about your mental health for any reason regardless of your score, please consult with a healthcare provider right away.

1. I have been able to laugh and see the funny side of things:
   a. As much as I always could (0)
   b. Not quite so much now (1)
   c. Definitely not so much now (2)
   d. Not at all (3)

2. I have looked forward with enjoyment to things:
    a. As much as I ever did (0)
    b. Rather less than I used to (1)
    c. Definitely less than I used to (2)
    d. Hardly at all (3)

3. I have blamed myself unnecessarily when things went wrong:
    a. Yes, most of the time (3)
    b. Yes, some of the time (2)
    c. Not very often (1)
    d. No, never (0)

4. I have been anxious or worried for no good reason:
    a. No, not at all (0)
    b. Hardly ever (1)
    c. Yes, sometimes (2)
    d. Yes, very often (3)

5. I have felt scared or panicky for no good reason:
    a. Yes, quite a lot (3)
    b. Yes, sometimes (2)
    c. No, not so much (1)
    d. No, not at all (0)

6. Things have been getting to me:
    a. Yes, most of the time I haven't been able to cope at all (3)

b. Yes, sometimes I haven't been coping as well as usual (2)
c. No, most of the time I have coped quite well (1)
d. No, I have been coping as well as ever (0)

7. I have been so unhappy that I have had difficulty sleeping:
   a. Yes, most of the time (3)
   b. Yes, sometimes (2)
   c. No, not very often (1)
   d. No, not at all (0)

8. I have felt sad or miserable:
   a. Yes, most of the time (3)
   b. Yes, quite often (2)
   c. Not very often (1)
   d. No, not at all (0)

9. I have been so unhappy that I have been crying:
   a. Yes, most of the time (3)
   b. Yes, quite often (2)
   c. Only occasionally (1)
   d. No, never (0)

10. The thought of harming myself has occurred to me:
    a. Yes, quite often (3)
    b. Sometimes (2)
    c. Hardly ever (1)
    d. Never (0)

PART 3

Reclaiming Postpartum

Prevention and Perspective

As always, there's more to the story. Even though postpartum health conditions are common among women who just gave birth, here are a few things I want you to know:

1. Postpartum health concerns also affect women who became mothers through different paths, apart from just carrying the baby themselves.
2. There are tangible steps that you can take to reduce your risk and support your well-being after becoming a mother.

3. The health implications of parenthood aren't all bad. In fact, mothers enjoy many health benefits that nonparents don't get to experience.

We will cover all these topics, and more, in detail in this section of the book.

CHAPTER 12

A Different Path to Motherhood

Jenna sat across from me, eyes wide and hopeful, waiting for my response. "So, what do you think?" she'd asked. As I started to answer, I moved my laptop aside so it wouldn't impede our conversation. In doing so, I knocked down the medication bottles she'd lined up on my desk after reading off the dosages so I could put them in her chart.

"Oh, sorry!" I exclaimed, climbing to the floor to pick them up and hand them back to her one at a time: Zyrtec, montelukast, prednisone, propranolol, Pepcid. The array included allergy medications, steroids, histamine-blocking medications, even antianxiety prescriptions. She'd tried name brand, off-brand, off-label usage. Yet none of them had helped. After the last prescription was safely returned to her purse, I sat back up, took a deep breath, and sighed.

"This is going to sound odd," I said, "but I think this is because of the IVF medications." Jenna's expression fell, and I knew why. First of all, she wasn't even taking any IVF medications anymore, and second, she didn't have any live children. I knew that bringing up the IVF was a sore spot for her. It was like a knife in a wound to suggest that the reason for her endless full-body hives was tied back to her failure to achieve the one thing that her heart had most desired, which was motherhood. But that wasn't all of it—I had now become yet another provider who had given another crazy-sounding answer as an explanation for her symptoms. See, Jenna had been told all kinds of things about her swollen face, rashes, and unbearable itching. Some said they were the result of allergies, which she'd never had before in her life; others, that it was just part of having Hashimoto's. One immunologist in particular told her that she "just has" chronic urticaria (aka chronic hives), which "just happens to some people," and that it will "just be part of her life now." Then there was me, saying that I believed her symptoms were the result of a failed procedure she'd endured over a year prior on a seemingly unrelated system of her body, which she couldn't undo even if she wanted to. Except it wasn't unrelated.

I explained to Jenna that even though she didn't walk away with a baby (or even a pregnancy) after enduring IVF, the hormone shifts involved in suppression of her cycle—like the stimulation of her ovaries, injection after injection of Lupron, estrogen priming, and progesterone shots—had effectively triggered many of the same hormonal environments that women go through during the early stages of pregnancy. It was those hormone shifts, regardless of the absence of pregnancy itself, that changed her immune function and caused the self-reactivity.

"Cue: hives, rashes, swelling. These immune symptoms are related to your thyroid, yes," I said, "but they're *mediated* by your other hormones. That's why they come and go."

"But I looked at my cycle," she replied, "and I've never once broken out when I'm on my period. How could it be my hormones?"

"You're right," I said. "But your period is when those hormone levels drop the lowest. Look here . . ." Just a few minutes prior, Jenna and I had written down the dates of both her several most recent periods and her few most recent outbreaks of hives. "See how each of these outbreaks falls around ten to twelve days before your period? You have irregular cycles because you're in perimenopause, so we can't count *after* your periods. You don't ovulate every month and sometimes don't ovulate at all. But when you do, you break out. The time between each breakout and your period is always about the same length as your luteal phase, the time between ovulation and your next period."

Jenna buried her face in her hands, and I quietly moved the box of tissues toward her. I knew that the emotion that had spring-loaded these tears was wrought by more than just a year of misdiagnosed hives, which frankly were bad enough on their own. For Jenna, it was also the trauma of IVF, the pain of infertility, the knowledge that now she was here in her forties, having tried and tried for a baby and walked away with an autoimmune disease instead. Without even so much as a positive pregnancy test, her hormones had cursed her with infertility and now a seemingly untreatable, unbearable rash. "It's like my body is literally fighting against me," she lamented.

Perhaps you're like Jenna, and your path to parenthood hasn't looked how you'd imagined it would. Maybe you, too, are dealing with empty arms and a full medication list without ever really having understood how you ended up here. Or maybe your own symptoms show a clear relationship to the timing of your parenthood journey, starting for the first time after an egg retrieval, a transfer that didn't take, or a miscarriage. Perhaps most confusing of all would be circumstances where the onset of symptoms matches perfectly to your entry into parenthood, but you became a mother through marriage, adoption, or surrogacy. Could it really be something more for you, too, or are you just tired because you have a child?

In situations like this, providers are more likely than ever to mistake concerning symptoms for normal experiences. If there's no baby or no pregnancy, both moms and doctors alike may miss the important time relationship where the answer to the symptoms is hiding. For as common as it is for doctors to overlook the risks for women with perfectly healthy babies conceived in a completely straightforward manner, greater still is the chance of misdiagnosis for women whose journeys to motherhood followed an atypical path.

You Don't Have to Experience Pregnancy to Experience "Postpartum" Health Risks

Have you ever heard of the concept of postpartum depression in fathers? In an article about the subject published by the University of Texas Southwestern Medical Center, experts state that new fathers experience overwhelm, sleep deprivation, and stress just like pregnant mothers and even experience hormonal shifts after their babies are born. In fact, as many as one in ten dads experience postpartum depression and anxiety.[1] While these rates are slightly lower than the average for postpartum depression among mothers who give birth, researchers have found that adoptive mothers face rates of depression that are equivalent or even greater,[2] ranging as high as 32 percent.[3]

These statistics speak to the widespread and complex nature of the relationship between parenthood and health. However, fathers and adoptive parents are not the only groups at risk of postpartum health concerns akin to those affecting birthing mothers. Let's take a moment to review the wide range of individuals who may experience post-parenthood health changes:

- **Adoptive parents:** From sleeplessness to the potential trauma of negative experiences with adoption agencies, financial strain, social factors, and even disappointment if adoption was not the first-choice parenthood plan, stress is a primary driver of health conditions in adoptive parents.
- **Mothers who gave up infants for adoption:** Even though mothers in these instances do not walk away with a child to parent, they still undergo the full breadth of physical and psychological shifts associated with pregnancy and postpartum. They also are much less likely to breastfeed or produce milk, therefore missing out on the protective benefits of lactation. They also carry the psychosocial trauma of infant separation.
- **Mothers experiencing chemical pregnancy, miscarriage, stillbirth, or termination:** Miscarriage refers to loss of a pregnancy during the first twenty weeks of gestation, but there are further classifications to

consider as well. The term *chemical pregnancy* is used to describe losses that occur prior to five weeks of gestation.[4] Many women themselves are unsure how to classify these experiences of loss so early in their pregnancy and, in my experience, may discount them as pregnancies at all. However, pregnancies that last even just a few days still bring about significant immunological and hormonal changes, even if a mother wasn't ever aware that she was pregnant. Likewise, we use the term *stillbirth* rather than *miscarriage* for pregnancies past twenty weeks gestation.[5] Similar to a miscarriage, stillbirth brings all the changes associated with pregnancy but for longer. Furthermore, stillbirth deliveries face a roughly 10 percent chance of C-section, which brings additional risks to the mother.[6]

- **Women who underwent unsuccessful fertility treatments:** Like with my patient Jenna, exposure to the medications involved in fertility treatments is often enough to trigger chronic health problems, even without ever achieving pregnancy. These include metabolic and hormonal changes,[7] and research shows that women who experience infertility even without achieving successful pregnancy face an increased risk of autoimmune disease.[8] Studies have also demonstrated that some of the medications necessary for IVF trigger changes to thyroid function, which are similar to the changes seen in pregnancy.[9]
- **Surrogate mothers:** These mothers experience all the same physical and psychological changes wrought by pregnancy with additional burdens associated with

infant separation. They also undergo additional exposures to medications and hormone treatments as an essential part of the IVF process. Research shows that surrogate mothers, so-called gestational carriers (a term that I feel detracts from the humanity of these women), face significantly increased risks of new-onset mental illness compared to mothers who themselves conceived with IVF or without intervention.[10]

- **Mothers who became parents through surrogacy:** Similar to adoptive parents, these mothers did not experience pregnancy as a means for parenting a particular child, but they likely attempted to do so prior. Some mothers may have undergone egg retrievals, which are invasive procedures used in surrogacy settings to create biologically related children. However, even with a donor or adoptive egg or embryo, mothers who become parents through surrogacy face similar experiences to adoptive parents.

Just like with postpartum women who recently delivered babies following pregnancy, doctors commonly overlook the health risks associated with these less-typical parenthood experiences for all the same reasons and more. For one, if the woman became a mother through adoption or through surrogacy, she may have never physically been involved in the creation of the pregnancy (such as with an egg donor, in the latter category). Therefore, the topic of parenthood's effect on her health may never come up in a medical appointment. But as we will discuss, health screening is not as simple as checking off a box that says "I have not given birth in the past twelve months." Then there's miscarriage and attempted but unsuccessful IVF cycles. I have yet to find a questionnaire that captures this detailed and highly individualized health history information. Many women don't share about miscarriages with their providers, especially if they happen early. Sadly, many doctors likewise don't ask. But a pregnancy is a pregnancy in the eyes of the immune system, the thyroid, and so many other commonly overlooked parts of the body. And that doesn't even take into account the stress of it all. Then, with situations like giving up a baby for adoption, carrying a pregnancy for the purpose of surrogacy, and termination, the complicated social, emotional, and physical factors bring additional layers of complexity. Of course, this is not ideal or recommended, but for reasons unique to the individual, some women may intentionally not disclose such aspects of their health history to providers for fear of judgment or ridicule or simply out of shame. When even the doctor isn't privy to the full knowledge of the patient's health history, the risk of misdiagnosis becomes even greater.

Parenthood-Related Health Problems Without Postpartum

We've already touched briefly on postpartum depression as it affects new parents, but mood changes are not the only health condition affecting individuals who have undergone circuitous, challenging, or distressing parenthood journeys. Let's take a closer look at some of them and explore how these experiences uniquely predispose women to developing health crises.

Mood Changes

Mood changes affect women who became parents through alternative means for many of the same reasons as women who develop depression, anxiety, and other disorders following pregnancy (no matter how long the pregnancy lasted, as we learned in chapter 11). Research has identified factors including expectations of oneself as a mother, the temperament of the child, social support, lack of rest, and preexisting mental health concerns, as well as interpersonal variables like bonding with the baby, marital satisfaction, and other forms of help (or lack thereof).[11] Additionally, women undergoing infertility treatments face higher rates of depression and anxiety, with as many as 40 percent of patients meeting the criteria for psychiatric diagnoses (typically anxiety and depression).[12] While every woman's journey is unique in the context of her own life, the stress and disappointment involved in trying to conceive, as well as the invasive nature of fertility treatments and their impact on the sexual relationship of marriage, are all clear contributing factors. My patients also often report spiritual struggles, feeling like their bodies failed them, or feeling broken.

These stories break my heart, but I also understand the sentiment behind them. At the end of the day, most parents would choose something other than these options (barring adoption, of course, which is a miracle in and of itself, and was always plan A for some families). Miscarriage, infertility, and loss of the opportunity to experience what you hoped your motherhood journey would look like are all possible sources of profound grief. My call to you, reader, is that if these circumstances describe you, don't think for one minute that you are not also deserving of the same care and support as any other mama. Please have the courage to reach out for support.

Nutrient Deficiencies

A few weeks after some family friends got the call that a baby had been placed in their home for adoption, I reached out to see how things were going. "I haven't eaten since yesterday morning, and I lost seven pounds this week, but we are so, so happy!" my friend replied. Aside from the hopefully obvious fact that adoptive parents need and benefit from meal trains, too, nutrient deficiencies easily arise in adoptive parents for many of the same reasons as they do in postpartum moms. While pregnancy and breastfeeding usually are not relevant concerns, the all-consuming nature of caring for a new child often leaves moms last in line for receiving the care they deserve. As parents, it's easy to overlook our own needs, no matter how old our children are or how they came to join our families. The "mom diet"—a dietary plan made up mostly of your child's leftovers—is not a sound nutritional strategy. New moms can easily develop nutrient deficiencies simply on account of the fact that overwhelm and hard work get in the way of balanced, nutritionally dense meals.

Furthermore, the blood loss accompanying miscarriage, plus the nutritional demands of pregnancy (even if it only lasted a short while) all contribute to depleted nutrient stores. And the body's nutritional needs increase during periods of stress,[13] a category that all types of parenthood, loss, and postpartum fall under, even if it's like my friend said, and you're "so, so happy!" Happiness doesn't mean you're well fed.

Autoimmune Disease

Do you remember Rachel from chapter 3? While the name was fictional, it represents the true story of a woman whose postpartum thyroiditis following a miscarriage went undiagnosed for far too long because doctors failed to recognize the relationship between her pregnancy, which ended tragically without a living child, and her autoimmune symptoms. Rachel's story was published as a case study in an academic journal in 2023, highlighting the importance of miscarriage as a possible trigger for autoimmune disease.

Stress and trauma are well-documented in scientific research as triggering events for new onset or worsening of autoimmune disease, including everything from inflammatory bowel disease to multiple sclerosis, lupus, Graves' disease, and more.[14] Loss of a child through miscarriage or even relinquishing a child through adoption or after acting as a surrogate for pregnancy are among the most stressful and traumatizing experiences possible in life. Loss and grief[15] and even caregiving are all cited as known triggers for autoimmune disease.[16] Whether it's traumatic stress, as in the case of pregnancy with child loss, or good stress in the form of caregiving, both are known to play a role in triggering autoimmune conditions, especially in women who have been touched by the stress of parenthood in unique ways.

Thyroid Disease

As we explored in chapter 6, the implications of pregnancy on thyroid health begin very early, as the pregnancy hormone hCG directly impacts thyroid function via brain feedback loops. So, whether the pregnancy lasts for nine months or nine days, whether or not it results in a live child, and whether or not that child comes home with the woman who delivered them does not matter. The thyroid is going to do what the thyroid is going to do, and sometimes it will not do what it should. Moreover, some IVF cycles involve the use of exogenous hCG hormone or a related hormone drug (known as a trigger shot) designed to help cue ovulation in a given time frame. Because of the direct effects of hCG on thyroid function, thyroid disorders may be triggered even if pregnancy was never achieved at all. This is relatively common among patients of mine, like Jenna, who never conceived despite undergoing the rigor and intensity of IVF and its associated medications.

Stress, such as that wrought by a circuitous parenthood experience, also plays a direct role in triggering thyroid disease for many people. The HPA axis, which we discussed in chapter 8, suppresses the brain functions responsible for regulating thyroid function.[17] There is also a profoundly abundant amount of research demonstrating the stress effects of thyroid-related disorders in particular.[18]

Adrenal Dysfunction

Speaking of stress, we know that chronic stress can trigger dysfunctional expressions of alarm in our nervous systems, producing debilitating symptoms that look a lot like "normal" postpartum. Well, no matter the path to parenthood, no matter how long you were (or weren't) pregnant, the stress of those experiences can cause health symptoms that look just like those of any other mother going through postpartum, whether or not you delivered a baby yourself and whether or not you are still holding that baby in your arms. Even though the symptoms of adrenal dysfunction in all three of its stages are caused by some degree of stress, they are not "just stress." We need to remember the complexity, the implications, and the true physiology behind these symptoms, no matter why or how motherhood came to be part of your story.

CHAPTER 13

A Healthy Postpartum Plan

Phew! I get it. We've covered a lot, and with how vulnerable the postpartum period makes us, it's easy to feel overwhelmed by what could go wrong after becoming a new mom. This chapter brings good news, finally. Although the hormonal and immunological shifts involved in childbirth and delivery can, and often do, trigger problematic health conditions, that doesn't necessarily have to become your reality. Moreover, you may not even experience the "normal" symptoms mimicked by these nutrient deficiencies, autoimmune disorders, thyroid problems, mental health conditions, and adrenal imbalances. There is so much that we can do to set ourselves up for a healthy postpartum so we can feel our very best as we step into the joys and challenges of parenthood. The following strategies are general health practices that I recommend to my patients as a prevention plan. Mama, I want you to know about them and use them too.

Strategy #1: Testing

As we have made abundantly clear throughout this book, you can't get an accurate diagnosis without specific and timely testing. Given that we're dealing with such a low standard of care for postpartum moms, most of us need to ask our providers directly for screening tests. In each of the previous five chapters, we outlined tests specific to each condition that can be used for early identification of concerning postpartum symptoms. The full list of tests and the testing cadence that I recommend are both summarized in appendix A of this book. Download the list to your phone or print it out and bring it with you to your appointments so you can advocate for yourself.

I'll keep this section short so as to not belabor a point that we've already dissected in detail. However, I also want to bring attention to one other important testing parameter we haven't covered: the importance of testing before and during pregnancy. Here's a question—have you ever had a provider offer you prenatal fertility testing? If not, you're not alone. In fact, I have never had a patient with this experience, either, at least outside of the functional medicine space. The setup of our nation's medical model makes such limited provision for preventive testing. I love when I have the opportunity to meet with women *before* they start trying to conceive because it gives us the chance to establish a baseline and set them up for success during the fertility, pregnancy, and postpartum journeys. As you'll see in appendix A, I recommend thorough testing before pregnancy as well as during. Recall from our conversation about thyroid disorders that 80 percent of women whose blood tests reveal elevated thyroid antibody levels in the third trimester of pregnancy go on to develop postpartum thyroiditis.[1] This statistic does no good if women can't implement any practical applications for themselves. Simply put, we need to test—early and often.

Strategy #2: Nutrition

The best way to prevent postpartum nutrient deficiencies and all the accompanying symptoms is to not have them prior to or during pregnancy. Moreover, the research has well established the link between dietary nutrient sufficiency and outcomes for fertility, pregnancy, and postpartum. For example, with preeclampsia, a complication of pregnancy and postpartum characterized by high blood pressure and protein in the urine, with risks of organ damage, stroke, and heart attack, consuming a mineral-rich diet high in selenium and vitamin D and low in ultra-processed foods has been shown to significantly reduce risk of developing this condition.[2] But it's not just postpartum preeclampsia that benefits from a well-rounded diet. Nutritional insufficiency, whether involving macronutrients (like carbohydrates, proteins, fats, and fiber) or micronutrients (like vitamins and minerals), has been shown to hold profound implications for adrenal function,[3] thyroid activity,[4] risk of postpartum mood disorders,[5] autoimmune disease,[6] and, of course, metabolic health.

Nutrition resources abound, so how should a postpartum mama eat to support her nutritional status and reduce risk of developing health problems? Here are a few general guidelines and specific recommendations for nutrient-dense foods that will serve as your postpartum allies.

General Nutritional Guidelines

- **Consume animal products abundantly:** I often refer to the work of nutrition researcher Ty Beal in my practice when educating patients about nutrition. Nutrient deficiency is a problem if a person either doesn't eat enough food in general (i.e., total calorie intake) or doesn't eat foods that have enough micronutrients per calorie. The best way to combat these problems is to eat a calorically abundant diet with a high density of micronutrients per calorie. In 2022, Ty Beal and Flaminia Ortenzi released a groundbreaking study detailing the micronutrient density of individual foods, identifying a list of items with the highest density and availability of micronutrients.[7] The list, in order, includes organ meats, small fish, dark green leafy vegetables, bivalves (clams, mussels, etc.), crustaceans, goat, beef, eggs, milk, canned fish with bones, mutton, and lamb. The researchers cited these as "foods to prioritize to fill common micronutrient gaps and reduce undernutrition."[8] With the exception of green leafy vegetables, everything on that list is animal based. Despite their popularity, plant-based protein sources, grains, nuts, and seeds did not make the list. This doesn't mean you can't or shouldn't consume those foods, but it does mean that if you want to avoid nutrient deficiencies without relying disproportionately on supplements, you need to eat animals.
- **Limit ultra-processed foods:** Just like a diet rich in whole foods from animal sources prevents nutrient deficiency, a diet in which ultra-processed, packaged

food products displace consumption of those foods increases risk of health problems. In fact, large-scale epidemiological studies have linked consumption of ultra-processed foods with risk of developing a host of interconnected cardiovascular and metabolic disorders, anxiety and depression, sleep disorders, as well as increased risk of dying *from all causes*.[9]

- **Hydrate:** Most sources recommend consuming half your body weight in ounces of water daily, and I agree, but with one caveat: If you're breastfeeding, you need to replace the water lost through lactation too. At a minimum, consume half your body weight plus number of ounces of breastmilk your baby consumes, which is usually estimated up to 36 oz daily at peak intake. For a 150-pound woman, this would be 75 oz plus 36 oz, or roughly 110 oz of water per day.
- **Limit caffeine:** I know—when you're not sleeping, you need to get energy somehow, especially if you have other children to care for. However, excessive caffeine intake can contribute to mental health issues, negatively impact sleep, and get in the way of your body's natural promptings to rest. I recommend limiting yourself to one six-ounce cup per day or the equivalent of no more than 150 mg of caffeine per day.

Specific Food Recommendations

A note before we get started on these: I recognize that postpartum is hard enough without worrying about groceries and cooking. Moreover, one of the most practical ways that friends and family members can offer help to a new mom is by bringing a meal. Please don't view this as a prescriptive list of the only foods to consume. Rather, when possible, add them into your diet as you are able. Additionally, many of these foods make sense to meal prep during pregnancy to get ready for postpartum, so consider making them ahead of time if you have the chance.

- **Bone broths:** Made from animal bones, which are rich in collagen, protein, and minerals, bone broths serve as a fantastic base for soups but also as a warm, soothing drink to sip on all day long. It's also a great source of hydration, can include electrolytes (when added), is a vehicle for healing herbs (see below), and can be prepared ahead of time, stored, and reheated as needed. I recommend consuming daily.
- **Slow-cooked meats and stews:** One of the best ways to get your daily intake of nutritious, nutrient-dense animal protein is through a "set and forget" slow cooker recipe. Like broths, the ingredients for stews and soups are easy to assemble in a freezer bag and prepare ahead of time. Slow-cooking meat increases its digestibility and reduces the burden of food preparation.[10] Consume daily.
- **Fish:** A fantastic source of micronutrients like selenium and zinc as well as minerals, omega-3s, and protein is low-toxin fish cuts like salmon, tilapia, sardines, anchovies, and trout. Sardines make a great substitute for tuna salad, but you can also find tinned varieties with peppers or tomato sauce, which are tasty on their own. Consider making a large portion of salmon once

per week, enjoying it hot and fresh for dinner, cold on a salad the next day, and mixed into a dip on day three.

- **Green leafy vegetables:** From fiber to folate, there are several reasons why greens like spinach and kale are high on Ty Beal's list. They blend easily into smoothies, cook down unobtrusively into soups and stews, and make mildly flavored, satisfying salads. Consume daily.
- **Herbs:** Many medicinal herbs with tremendous health benefits are also widely used for culinary purposes. Research demonstrates that many herbs support health in all seasons of life, including with blood sugar regulation, weight management, digestion, cognitive function, inflammation control, and more. These include chili pepper, cinnamon, ginger, black pepper, turmeric, fenugreek, rosemary, and garlic.[11] I recommend consuming these abundantly in teas, soups, and other recipes.

Strategy #3: Exercise

Most resources recommend against exercising until receiving the "all clear" from an obstetric provider at the six-week follow-up appointment. While I am a huge advocate for rest (see strategy #4), I also disagree based on the definition of exercise. We often think of exercise as a means for weight loss, requiring dedicated effort, an elevated level of intensity, and sufficient strain (you know, "no pain, no gain"). Well, I want to challenge you to also consider breath work, slow stretching, and gentle calisthenics aimed at stability as under the umbrella of exercise and to consider utilizing them right away. Most of these are best employed under the supervision of a pelvic floor physical therapist, but many can be completed easily and safely at home. Consider the following exercises with the goals of restoring stability, preventing injury, and rehabilitating the body after the physical trauma of labor. Complete several sets of ten reps each day.

- **Belly breathing/360-degree breathing:** When taking a breath, the diaphragm muscle should contract downward, allowing your lower abdomen to relax and expand. Meanwhile, your chest and the muscles of your shoulders and ribs should not move at all.
- **Pelvic floor coordination:** When inhaling, the pelvic floor should remain relaxed. Upon exhalation, the pelvic floor should contract and stabilize. For lack of a better visualization, imagine your vagina "sucking upward," as if through a straw. Make sure to relax completely with each inward breath.
- **Transversus abdominis (TVA) breathing/contraction:** Also known as "hug the baby," activating this band of muscles found in the triangular area between the hip bones and pubic bone provides stabilization to prevent injury. Imagine "zipping up" your abdomen from your pubic bone to your sternum on each exhale, with your belly button moving straight back toward your spine.
- **Glute squeezes and (eventually) glute bridges:** This is a gentle method for restrengthening your glute muscles and retraining your brain to engage these stability muscles during movement. Complete each movement

while simultaneously activating the TVA upon exhalation. Perform this exercise while lying on your back with knees bent and feet flat on the floor about twelve inches apart.

- **Chin retractions:** Due to poor core stability following pregnancy, many women develop a pattern of holding their heads forward while standing. Spend time lying on a flat surface with knees bent and feet flat on the floor. Simultaneously draw the chin backward toward the floor while imagining a string attached to the top of your head is pulling your head to lengthen your neck and spine.
- **Full-body stretches:** Utilize arm circles, a lunge stretch, hip extensions, cobra, child's pose, and other passive, gentle stretches for each muscle and joint of your body every day.
- **Walking:** As your body allows, complete several ten- to fifteen-minute walks per day (or whatever is comfortable for you and does not leave any part of your body sore) as soon as you are comfortable following delivery. Please note that if you cannot sustain this level of activity by one week postpartum, it is a sign of a deeper health problem.

Strategy #4: Rest

To recover from a lack of sleep, you need more sleep than simply the number of hours that you missed. There is no algorithm or mathematic equation for exactly how much, but consider this: We need sleep and rest to maintain our health.

Lack of sleep is not just a lost opportunity for needed recovery but also an added stressor (à la chapter 8). So, combining labor (which often disrupts sleep) with frequent nighttime newborn wakings and the physical stress of delivery, we enter motherhood with a major deficit. This means we need *more than* nine hours of sleep to protect our health, especially if that sleep is interrupted. We need to take a break from physical and mental strain and give our minds and bodies the opportunity for deep rest. Consider these strategies for supporting your rest, if possible:

- **Enlist help:** Write down all the people you can think of who can help you postpartum, and make a list of things they can help you with. Everything from dishes to laundry to cleaning can be outsourced, and you can also ask for help with caring for your other children, if applicable. Plan early to get your support system in place. Hired help is also available in the form of postpartum doulas, nannies, and other household services. If people in your life are a limited resource, don't forget about things like paper plates and grocery delivery! These conveniences may not be your first choice, but they can play a huge role in helping you adjust to life with a new baby.
- **Do just one thing per day:** Remember the advice I shared at the very beginning of the book? Caring for a newborn is a full-time, round-the-clock job, and all the other responsibilities of daily life need to take a break in order to support your recovery. For at least the first week, I really don't recommend doing

anything other than short walks and meeting your basic needs. But after that, consider completing just one chore or errand per day, whether that be laundry, a pediatrician visit, or a trip to the park with your older children. Only once such chores and errands no longer leave you feeling more tired than you were beforehand should you expand the intensity or length of such responsibilities.

- **Rest when the baby rests:** This is my own adaptation of the old adage "sleep when the baby sleeps," as it's not always possible or necessary to be completely asleep every time your baby is. However, if the baby is sleeping, you should at least be resting, which means sitting, reclining, lying down, napping, or generally taking a break. Resist the urge to do chores while the baby is napping, at least until you are no longer fatigued from them.

Strategy #5: Detox

Following pregnancy, the body works hard to get rid of old, broken-down hormones, immune molecules, inflammatory chemicals, and waste. The blood supply slowly shrinks back down to prepregnancy levels, which means the body needs to eliminate old red blood cells and metabolic byproducts. We already touched on hydration and good nutrition, which are both essential factors for supporting healthy detoxification, but here are a few other strategies to keep in mind to support postpartum recovery:

- **Eat fiber:** Fiber passes through the digestive system without absorbing into our bloodstream. In doing so, it brings waste products with it to clear them away. Fiber bulks up stool, preventing constipation and hemorrhoids; helps avoid straining, which may injure the pelvic floor; and binds to everything from excess estrogen[12] to cholesterol.[13] It also improves blood sugar regulation.[14] Aim for at least 35 g per day from fresh vegetables. While supplements can be helpful, they are more likely to cause adverse side effects and don't come with the added nutrition that whole foods do.

- **Limit toxin exposure:** Our bodies are working hard enough as it is to recover from pregnancy, and we can help them with their efforts by reducing our exposure to toxins like pesticides, food additives, fragrance chemicals, harmful chemicals added to personal hygiene products (e.g., phthalates, parabens), alcohol, plastic, and heavy metals found in cookware and food storage containers.
- **Get some sunlight:** Intermittent, safe sunlight exposure, particularly in the morning, triggers vitamin D production, which naturally helps the liver metabolize and break down toxins, including some medications.[15] It also regulates mood and circadian rhythm[16] to promote deep sleep, which is how the brain detoxifies.[17] Spending time in sunlight is also a low-exertion method of inducing sweating, another of the body's natural detox mechanisms.[18]

Strategy #6: Controlling Stress

Stress plays such a major role in the onset of nearly all the conditions we discussed in this book, which are commonly mistaken as normal. But it also plays a role in countless other postpartum conditions that we haven't even touched on! Stress management is foundational for recovery and health as you adjust to motherhood with a new little one in your family. Keep these strategies in mind, whether you're facing new stressors, coping with existing ones, or simply putting together a toolbox for yourself to support your well-being. Keep in mind that the above strategies, including nutrition, rest, and gentle exercise, also help maintain manageable workloads and keep stress levels low.

- **Work with a therapist:** I recommend counseling for nearly everyone. This is not because I think everyone has a diagnosable mental health disorder but rather because intense life transitions like bringing another child into the world are inherently challenging. Mental health providers help you cultivate effective and healthy coping strategies and build a foundation for personal wellness in light of the sacrifices inherent to parenting.
- **Consider support groups:** Outside of the joys of meeting and loving your new baby, infants often bring their own health challenges, which can add stress. Breastfeeding difficulties, colic, sleep struggles, and more can be helped by social support from others who *get it*. Sometimes, even the most supportive partners are not enough to provide the necessary camaraderie or wisdom to be truly helpful in these circumstances. We were made to live in community!

- **Utilize mindfulness and meditation:** Commit to taking postpartum one day at a time. The sheer amount of work involved in caring for a newborn itself can weigh on even the hardiest mama. That being said, things change fast. To help keep yourself grounded and present, consider a mindfulness, prayer, or meditation practice.
- **Slow down your pace:** Are you rushing around trying to get things done, acting like a tiger is chasing you? As moms, sometimes that is our default mode. My challenge for you, instead, is to intentionally slow down your pace of moving, speaking, and intention. Give yourself permission to go at exactly the pace you need to in order to remain relaxed.
- **Avoid multitasking:** Similar to rushing through a set of tasks, multitasking adds stress because it doesn't actually work. Rather than effectively doing two things at once, it's been found that the brain instead rapidly switches back and forth between the two tasks, which is akin to a two-for-one deal of mental rushing and constant interruption.[19]
- **Pay attention to your triggers:** You will likely have a lower tolerance for stressors than you did previously, and that is to be expected. Between the hormone shifts and sleeplessness, little things can easily put you over the edge because your bucket is already so full during the postpartum time. However, these triggers are going to vary for everyone. Take note of what makes you feel stressed and validate those feelings even if the same situations never used to bother you before. For

example, you might never have been bothered by your dog's barking, but now between a sleeping baby and sensory overload, it puts you over the edge. Could you consider a dog walker, doggy daycare, or deactivating your doorbell for a while to reduce provocation? Consider which little changes you can make to protect your peace. Trust me, those little things can go a long way so that you have more capacity for the bigger, more important stressors.

At the end of the day, we can't prevent every single health problem. However, having a plan in place to protect your nervous system and establishing a foundation for your basic needs will help you discern what to do about symptoms when they pop up. Following these guidelines will mitigate how much postpartum experiences negatively impact your quality of life. In other words, if the symptoms really are normal, this self-care blueprint will help alleviate them (because postpartum should be enjoyable, not a form of slow suffering!) These strategies also help reduce the risk of developing true health problems, like nutrient deficiencies or adrenal dysfunction, and support your body in making healthy hormonal transitions. If you implement all these principles and still notice persistent symptoms, you know it's time to get checked out and not leave your provider's office until you have a plan in place to figure out the root cause. Taking care of yourself is not only your right but also a gift to your baby by helping you become the healthiest person you can be.

CHAPTER 14

What About the Good?

After reading a book like this, you might find yourself on high alert. You're motivated to advocate for yourself and armed with both vigilance and a plan to make sure you remain healthy. But perhaps a part of you struggles to wrap your mind around the risks of motherhood. Most conversations center around the joys of meeting a new baby but also the hardships of adjusting to the diapers, the crying, the breastfeeding challenges. We know that the powerful love of bringing a new baby into the world makes it all worth it, but is each subsequent child just going to detract further from your health?

This is where I want to come in with what I hope is a breath of fresh air. For one, knowledge of what *could* go wrong is a means for equipping you to care for yourself, not something to be afraid of or a reason not to grow your family. Just like there are risks to pregnancy and childbirth, postpartum also brings some risks. But knowledge of those risks and having a game plan will help you keep those risks from becoming a reality or, as many women unfortunately experience, prevent those risks from becoming a health condition that goes undiagnosed for years and years.

That being said, many women—most, even—go on to have healthy pregnancies and postpartum experiences. What's more, on a physiological level, childbirth, breastfeeding, and parenting all actually bring tremendous benefits to parents. With perks like reduced cancer risks, increased longevity, and better subjective reports of quality of life, there are actually more benefits than risks for mamas. We're going to explore a handful of them in this chapter. So, take a deep breath, remember that even though our bodies face unique threats on account of carrying our babies inside our bodies, we also bear the privilege of doing that in the first place, along with countless physiological benefits that will accompany us through the remainder of our lives. That is, all in addition to the tremendously purpose-filled and sanctifying gift of loving, caring for, and bringing up a child.

Motherhood Increases Longevity

Children are truly a gift that keeps on giving, as data shows that bringing new life into the world begets longer life for mothers. Epidemiological studies demonstrate that women who are mothers have a lower risk of dying from any cause, and an overall increased life expectancy compared to women who have never had children. According to one 2017 study, mothers live an estimated 1.5 years longer than their childfree counterparts.[1] As we will discuss later, having children reduces a mother's risk of developing certain chronic diseases, but she is also less likely to die from those diseases. A study among elderly individuals living in Australia found that regardless of an existing diagnosis of high blood pressure, diabetes, or being overweight, risk of dying from these diseases decreased proportionately to the number of children each mother had.[2] In other words, the more, the better! Another study in Ireland showed the same thing—that as the number of children increased, risk of dying decreased, regardless of the overall health status of that mother.[3]

Interestingly, in these studies, the hypothesis that women who are mothers engage in more health-promoting lifestyle behaviors does not explain the increase in longevity. In fact, some studies even showed that women with children are more likely to smoke and become overweight, less likely to exercise, and more likely to suffer from back pain.[4] They also are more likely to develop some of those chronic diseases, particularly those related to metabolism and insulin resistance; they just are not as likely to die from them. So, what explains the benefit?

The current best explanation for increased longevity associated with childbearing comes down to the role of estrogen. Estrogen exposure is overall higher in women who have delivered children, for two reasons. First, estrogen levels skyrocket during pregnancy, which accounts for nine to ten months of heightened estrogen exposure for each full-term pregnancy. Second, pregnancy and childbirth appear to delay the onset of menopause.[5] Later menopause translates to a greater total number of menstrual cycles, estrogen and all, in a given woman's lifetime. Between the pregnancies themselves and the delay in cessation of menstruation, women who have children have proportionately greater estrogen exposure per number of births.

Estrogen's role in longevity is not well understood, but a 2016 study found a link between estrogen exposure and telomere length.[6] Telomeres are parts of our DNA that play a role in cellular regeneration and aging. All of our cells have lifespans, but telomeres influence how many times those cells are able to regenerate after they die. In other words, aging and longevity are a reflection of how likely our cells are to regenerate themselves so that our whole body can live longer. It's a microscopic-to-macroscopic translation of aging. Well, the good news for women with children is that higher estrogen exposure throughout their lives protects those telomeres, keeping them longer. This, in turn, allows the woman's cells to regenerate a greater number of times, increasing the chances that she will live a long life and decreasing the chances of dying for any reason!

Aging and longevity are complex subjects, and there is certainly more to the story than just estrogen. In fact, there is so much to the story that researchers have not been able to fully explain all of the reasons why pregnancy and parenthood extend life—especially considering that even fathers have been found to live longer because of parenthood, and they certainly can't thank high estrogen levels for their longevity. However, I want to highlight the estrogen here, because even though hormone shifts associated with pregnancy may trigger health risks, as we discussed in all the previous chapters of this book, they also offer us benefits. It's truly a puzzling paradox!

Motherhood Decreases Disease Risks

There's more good news to behold, as not only do mothers live longer than child-free women, but they also are more likely to be healthier in some ways. While pregnancy and childbearing do carry increased risks of certain hormonal and immune system diseases (many of which are treatable), these life experiences also decrease the risk of developing a number of other illnesses, generally increasing quality of life while enjoying longevity along the way.

One of the most marked risk reductions comes in the form of cancer—of a variety of types. Women with children are 72.5 percent less likely to die from any type of cancer than women without children.[7] The overall risk varies by cancer variety, but as a whole, this is a huge benefit to women's health in the realm of pregnancy. The clearest and most direct benefit comes in terms of endometrial cancer risk. Researchers found that women who have ever carried a full-term pregnancy enjoy a 41 percent lower risk of developing endometrial cancer, and each subsequent pregnancy reduces the risk by approximately 15 percent.[8] Even pregnancies that never reach full term demonstrate some reduced risk, attributable to the presence of progesterone.

Ovarian cancer risks also decrease proportionately with number of children birthed. Women who have never had children face a 24 percent greater risk of developing this disease compared to women with one child. Each additional child offers a further 6 percent reduction in risk, and breastfeeding offers further benefit. For each year of breastfeeding, women enjoy a 10 percent reduced risk of ovarian cancer.[9] Breastfeeding also dramatically reduces risk of developing breast cancer, which is the most common cancer among women.[10] For every twelve months of breastfeeding, risk of breast cancer drops by 4.3 percent in addition to the 7 percent decreased risk for each birth.[11] Breastfeeding even decreases the risk of cancer in carriers of the BRCA1 gene mutation, which is considered one of the most significant risk factors for development of aggressive breast cancers, by up to 55 percent.[12] Doing a little math here, if a woman gives birth to three children—just one more than the (rough) average of two per household in the United States, and breastfeeds each child for the full recommended two years, her risk of developing breast cancer drops by 46.8 percent, which is nearly half.

Here's a question to contend with: Rates of breast, ovarian, and endometrial cancer are rising. Is it because women today are having fewer children, and are less likely to breastfeed those children, than they were one hundred years ago?

The benefits abound for more than just cancer risks. Studies show that women with children face only 34 percent of the risk of dying from heart disease that childfree women do and only 53 percent of the risk of dying from infection.[13] Again, we don't fully understand the mechanism behind these phenomena, but it's a benefit and a gift nonetheless.

Motherhood Improves Mental Health

I don't know about you, but in my book, children are more costly than anything. They cost our finances, our time, our bodies. But what makes it all worth it, and what outweighs these costs beyond any shadow of a doubt, is the joy, meaning, and purpose that they bring to our lives. Love and its many benefits can't truly be measured in hours, lab results, dollars, or anything else. I love my kids for all the millions of little things that make them who they are but also because of how much they fill my heart and improve my quality of life. Well, the statistics agree with this sentiment: Women with children enjoy better mental health throughout their lives than those without, even factoring in the risks of postpartum mood disorders.

Before we dive into some of these details, I want to make clear that while the US population carries high rates of postpartum depression, this is a specific type of mood disorder that is unique to the postpartum period and is highly treatable with conservative, holistic, supportive health strategies. It is unique compared to other types of depression, especially major depressive disorder, and does not necessarily translate to increased risk of other mood disorders throughout life. Rather, pregnancy and childbirth are ultimately protective of mental health when considering mood from the perspective of longevity and overall reported quality of life.

In fact, many of the benefits of parenting on mental health can be seen within five years of giving birth. A study conducted in first-time mothers showed that on average their mental health demonstrated overall improvements following childbirth compared to prior (when assessed twice annually for five years before and after childbirth).[14] These longer-term trends are important when evaluating the risk of depression in the postpartum period compared to life thereafter.

Over the course of a lifespan, women who have children face a lower overall risk of developing major depression, with even greater benefits with subsequent children. A population study of over five hundred thousand women found that women experienced a 9 percent reduced risk of developing major depression for each child they had.[15] While this study was completed on Chinese rather than American women, the sheer magnitude of the linear relationship between children and mental health—in combination with the fact that the same response was not seen in fathers—indicates a mechanism dependent on the fact of pregnancy itself.

Longer, Happier, Healthier Lives

Anyone who has ever entered into motherhood knows that child-rearing is no walk in the park (despite how many literal walks you might take in a park throughout a given week). There is sacrifice involved, and sometimes the toll taken on your health in the immediate aftermath of pregnancy and postpartum can feel so extremely daunting. Especially if you've been dealing with debilitating symptoms and struggling to get an accurate diagnosis (and, subsequently, effective healthcare), you may find yourself wondering if the hardship will ever end. Well, the good news is that it will. As soon as you are able to get the help you deserve, you will see just how bright of a future that sweet little baby will bring you.

From decreased cancer and cardiovascular risks and an overall decreased risk of dying from any particular condition, paired with an overall extended lifespan with increased markers for mental health, parenthood really does deliver more than it takes. This doesn't detract from the hard work involved, but it does prove that it's not all for naught. Realizing all the ways that postpartum can go awry might paint a seemingly grim picture for the future. But just because postpartum healthcare in our country is in tremendous need of reform doesn't mean that there isn't hope on the horizon for a future that far outshines the magnitude of today's struggles.

As this book comes to a close, I want you to remember, dear mama, that your body was made good—ultimately. Any of the disruptions or dysfunctions that may arise postpartum pale in comparison to the tremendous gift that your baby is to your family, your heart, and even to the physical health of your body. What a blessing indeed!

Conclusion

Part of the reality of working in medicine is that I am personally more aware of the health experiences of the people in my community than the average person. This is obviously due to the fact that I am paid by my patients for the precise purpose of listening to their health concerns, and a substantial portion of my week every week is dedicated to doing exactly that. But it's also because the people in my personal life willingly disclose details about their health to me that they just don't share as readily with others. I mean, it makes sense—they certainly aren't going to ask me to help them with computer programming (they'll ask their tech-savvy friend about that). Rather, they know I speak the language of medicine, and so I am their go-to person for asking health-related questions or lamenting medical woes.

In my years of listening to such health experiences from my own friends and family, it struck me one day that every single woman in my life who is a mother has experienced a postpartum health challenge. Some of them were acute problems, even emergencies, which their doctors readily recognized and treated. But many others were, like me, dismissed by their doctors. While they went on to eventually get a diagnosis, it sometimes wasn't until years after the symptoms first started. Again, like me, none of their medical providers volunteered any follow-up care or screenings apart from the six-week postpartum visit (and maybe a depression questionnaire). Instead, they had to do their own digging and advocate for themselves to get help. This is all despite the decades of medical research outlining the relationship between pregnancy and new-onset health conditions postpartum.

The scientists know about it. The doctors theoretically know about it (after all, I learned all of this in school). And still, the policies and standards of care have yet to catch up. Nobody is even talking about it! Instead, the cries for help are met with "Welcome to the club" and "Your six-week follow-up is all clear, see you in a year!" As we know, a lot can happen in a year.

Well, my hope for this book is to change that. Mama, you deserve better care. You deserve thorough, proactive screening. You deserve for your provider to put the pedal to the metal when it comes to medical research and maternal health, to be several steps ahead of you to ensure the best possible outcomes and quality of life. Granted, such a macrolevel of change will probably take a long time. But until then, you have the pages of this book as your ally.

If you haven't yet given birth, you now know how to plan accordingly. As they say, an ounce of prevention is worth a pound of cure.

If you're already postpartum and not sure how to know if your experiences are normal, you have a toolbox at the ready to help you get the proactive healthcare you deserve.

If your baby has arrived and you can clearly see that you're struggling, my hope is that this book gives *you* hope that such a state of suffering is not your new normal.

If you're a loved one of a new or expecting mama, you likewise now have a talking point or resource to gently point them in the right direction to get help.

If you work in healthcare yourself, you are uniquely positioned to speak into the lives of women and point them in the right direction. Even if other healthcare providers—including the ones who are arguably responsible for facilitating such preventive care—are not having these conversations, you can start them. Whether you are a provider in another field or a worker in the healthcare field but not directly overseeing patient care, *share what you've learned.* You never know who might be needing your help. (Which, odds are, is probably everyone.)

Ladies, we're in this together. They say it takes a village, and I am now part of your village as it relates to your health. But I can't reach through the pages of this book to perform an exam or write a lab test order for you. Instead, you're going to need to speak up. Whether that means talking to your own doctor, gently nudging a friend in the right direction, sharing your own experience in a public way, or whatever else you need to do, help spread the word. Postpartum is such a vulnerable time, and I know how valuable all those little bits of help and encouragement have been to me along the way as I have navigated my own postpartum journeys. Your voice matters!

As we part ways, I want to leave with a few additional encouragements. First, the good news about all of the health conditions outlined in this book is that they are treatable. There is help available, which includes a variety of options that you can choose from to support your well-being in the way that makes the most sense for your life and values. Second, even if this is a challenging time in your health journey and your life, don't forget to celebrate the good. Your baby and the experience of motherhood are such gifts. Find ways to celebrate this truth even while you navigate health struggles because, as with all hard things, *this too shall pass*.

And finally, remember that you are not alone. You are not the first and won't be the last to face struggles exactly like what you are facing today. Reach out for help, whether that be from a doctor, a friend, a family member, a counselor, or a mentor. It is in the community and camaraderie of motherhood that we find healing.

In health,
Dr. Alexandra MacKillop, DC

Acknowledgments

Postpartum moms need better care. I know this because of my own experiences bringing children into the world, but more importantly because of the thousands of stories shared with me by my patients who have faced similar health struggles, have wrestled with the same types of questions, and have likewise needed to advocate for themselves in the midst of total overwhelm. I want to take this opportunity to thank these women for their vulnerability, for their trust in me as a provider, and for their courage to seek help—all of which have inspired and encouraged me to write this book. *The Postpartum Check-In* would not exist if not for all of you. I do not have words for the tremendous privilege it is to touch the lives of others in this way.

On that note, I also want to thank you, my readers. Writing is one of my favorite ways to communicate, to create, and to share what's on my heart. Thank you for making that possible.

Thank you also to all the others who helped this book come to be, both directly and indirectly:

To Keely, my agent—I appreciate your support, attention, encouragement, and guidance so very much. Thank you for believing in me as a writer and allowing me the chance to bring my words to print.

To Andrea, my incredible editor, and the team at Revell—it has been such a blessing to work with you. Thank you for your support of this project, for sharing your expertise, and for partnering with me to bring this message to the world. I have learned so much from you and am so grateful for the opportunities that you have afforded me.

To Linda—thank you for all your encouragement and advice along the way. Thank you for sharing your experience and for giving me a sense of community in the world of writing, which feels lonely at times.

To my family—my children, who gave me the role of Mama, which is my greatest privilege and honor; my husband, who supports me in every imaginable way; and my sister, who believes in me before I believe in myself.

And I thank God, the creator of the universe and everything in it. Somehow, you hold all of these broken things together.

APPENDIX A

Lab Testing

Recommended Laboratory Testing Cadence

The following lab tests are usually included as part of an annual wellness examination. I recommend they all be completed:

1. Prior to pregnancy, if possible
2. During the first trimester of pregnancy
3. During the third trimester of pregnancy
4. Six weeks postpartum
5. Between three and six months postpartum
6. Between nine and twelve months postpartum

Routine Postpartum Labs

- Complete blood count (CBC)
- Comprehensive metabolic panel (CMP)

- Hemoglobin A1c
- Fasting insulin
- Thyroid panel, including thyroid-stimulating hormone (TSH), free and total T3, free and total T4, and thyroglobulin (Tg)/thyroid peroxidase (TPO) antibodies
- Morning cortisol
- Iron, ferritin, and total iron binding capacity (TIBC)
- Zinc serum
- Magnesium, red blood cell (RBC)
- Vitamin D
- Vitamin B_{12}/folate
- OmegaCheck (omega-3 and -6 fatty acids)

Postpartum Visit Cadence (with Any Provider, Minimum)

1. Two weeks postpartum check-in/visit
2. Six weeks postpartum visit (regularly scheduled)
3. At least ten sessions of pelvic floor physical therapy (to be completed within the first year)
4. Quarterly wellness visits for the first year postpartum (with any provider)
5. Appointments with all providers previously seen before pregnancy at least once in the first year postpartum

APPENDIX B

Resources

Drugs and Lactation Database (LactMed) for Drug Safety While Breastfeeding
https://www.ncbi.nlm.nih.gov/books/NBK501922/

Find a Board-Certified Lactation Consultant
https://iblce.org/

Find a DONA Certified Doula or Postpartum Doula
https://www.dona.org/what-is-a-doula-2/find-a-doula/

Find a Functional Medicine Certified Provider
https://www.ifm.org/find-a-practitioner

Find a Myofunctional Therapist for Breastfeeding Support and Tongue Tie Evaluation
https://www.myofunctionaltherapists.com/

Find a Pelvic Rehabilitation Provider
https://hermanwallace.com/

Find a Bradley Method Birth Class Instructor
https://www.bradleybirth.com/directory.aspx

National Maternal Mental Health Hotline
1-833-TLC-MAMA

Spinning Babies Prenatal Support
https://www.spinningbabies.com/

Work with Dr. Alexandra MacKillop, DC
AlexandraMacKillop.com

Notes

Chapter 2 Postpartum Is Forever

1. F. E. Hytten, "Blood Volume Changes in Normal Pregnancy," *Clinics in Haematology* 14, no. 3 (1985): 601–12, https://pubmed.ncbi.nlm.nih.gov/4075604/.

2. Shikha Singh, "Thyroid Disease and Pregnancy," in *StatPearls* (StatPearls Publishing, 2025), https://www.ncbi.nlm.nih.gov/books/NBK538485/.

3. Noel M. Lee and Sumona Saha, "Nausea and Vomiting of Pregnancy," *Gastroenterology Clinics of North America* 40, no. 2 (2011): 309–34, https://www.ncbi.nlm.nih.gov/pmc/articles/PMC3676933/.

4. Jodi L. Pawluski et al., "Serotonin and Motherhood: From Molecules to Mood," *Frontiers in Neuroendocrinology* 55 (April 2019): 100768, https://www.ncbi.nlm.nih.gov/pmc/articles/PMC6541513/.

5. Robert Martone, "Scientists Discover Children's Cells Living in Mothers' Brains," *Scientific American*, December 4, 2012, https://www.scientificamerican.com/article/scientists-discover-childrens-cells-living-in-mothers-brain/.

6. Leanne Duthie and Rebecca M. Reynolds, "Changes in the Maternal Hypothalamic-Pituitary-Adrenal Axis in Pregnancy and Postpartum: Influences on Maternal and Fetal Outcomes," *Neuroendocrinology* 98, no. 2 (2013): 106–15, https://doi.org/10.1159/000354702.

Chapter 3 How and Why Healthcare Providers Get It Wrong

1. James R. Kang et al., "Postpartum Thyroiditis Mimicking Central Hypothyroidism: The Perfect Thyming," *Cureus* 15, no. 7 (July 28, 2023): e42630, https://doi.org/10.7759/cureus.42630.

2. Eric J. Topol, "Toward the Eradication of Medical Diagnostic Errors," *Science* 383, no. 6681 (2024): 1234–35, https://doi.org/10.1126/science.adn9602.

3. Nicole M. Krenitsky et al., "Diagnostic Errors in Obstetric Morbidity and Mortality: Methods for and Challenges in Seeking Diagnostic Excellence," *Journal of Clinical Medicine* 13, no. 14 (2024): 4245, https://doi.org/10.3390/jcm13144245.

4. Zhimin Poon et al., "Experiences of Primary Care Physicians Managing Postpartum Care: A Qualitative Research Study," *BMC Family Practice* 22 (2021): 139, https://doi.org/10.1186/s12875-021-01494-w.

5. "Weill Cornell Medicine and NewYork-Presbyterian Receive NIH Support for Project Addressing Postpartum Maternal Health in Underserved Communities," *Weill Cornell Medicine Newsroom*, September 6, 2023, https://news.weill.cornell.edu/news/2023/09/weill-cornell-medicine-and-newyork-presbyterian-receive-nih-support-for-project.

6. Diorella Lopez-Gonzalez and Anil Kopparapu, "Postpartum Care of the New Mother," in *StatPearls* (StatPearls Publishing, 2022).

7. "Postpartum Thyroiditis," American Thyroid Association, updated September 2023, https://www.thyroid.org/postpartum-thyroiditis.

8. Kristian Tore Jørgensen et al., "Childbirths and Risk of Female Predominant and Other Autoimmune Diseases in a Population-Based Danish Cohort," *Journal of Autoimmunity* 38, no. 2–3 (2011), https://doi.org/10.1016/j.jaut.2011.06.004.

9. Sybil G. Dessie et al., "Do Obstetrical Providers Counsel Women About Postpartum Pelvic Floor Dysfunction?" *Journal of Reproductive Medicine* 60, no. 5–6 (2015): 205–10, https://pubmed.ncbi.nlm.nih.gov/26126305/.

10. Nancy Byatt et al., "Building Obstetric Provider Capacity to Address Perinatal Depression Through Online Training," *Journal of Women's Health* 30, no. 10 (2021): 1452–60, https://doi.org/10.1089/jwh.2020.8843.

11. Diana Ramos, "What to Expect at a Postpartum Checkup—And Why the Visit Matters," *American College of Obstetricians and Gynecologists*, updated February 2024, https://www.acog.org/womens-health/experts-and-stories/the-latest/what-to-expect-at-a-postpartum-checkup-and-why-the-visit-matters.

12. Hannah T. Neprash et al., "Measuring Primary Care Exam Length Using Electronic Health Record Data," *Medical Care* 59, no. 1 (2021): 62–66, https://doi.org/10.1097/MLR.0000000000001450.

13. American College of Obstetricians and Gynecologists, "ACOG Committee Opinion No. 736: Optimizing Postpartum Care," *Obstetrics & Gynecology* 131, no. 5 (2018): 140–50, https://doi.org/10.1097/AOG.0000000000002633.

14. "Postpartum Thyroiditis," American Thyroid Association, https://www.thyroid.org/postpartum-thyroiditis/.

15. Bonnie Rochman, "Why France Pays for Postpartum Women to 'Re-Educate' Their Vagina," *TIME*, February 22, 2012, https://healthland.time.com/2012/02/22/why-france-pays-for-postpartum-women-to-re-educate-their-vagina/.

16. Janet W. Rich-Edwards et al., "Does Pregnancy Alter Life-Course Lipid Trajectories? Evidence from the CARDIA Study," *Journal of Clinical Endocrinology & Metabolism* 105, no. 2 (2020): e378–e386, https://doi.org/10.1210/clinem/dgz157.

17. Christine M. Guardino et al., "Chronic Stress and C-Reactive Protein in Mothers During the First Postpartum Year," *Psychosomatic Medicine* 79, no. 4 (2017): 450–60, https://doi.org/10.1097/PSY.0000000000000424.

18. Zhongzheng Niu et al., "Association of Breastfeeding Duration with 12-Month Postpartum Blood Lipids in a Predominantly Lower-Income Hispanic Pregnancy Cohort in Los Angeles," *International Journal of Environmental Research and Public Health* 19, no. 5 (2022): 3008, https://doi.org/10.3390/ijerph19053008.

Chapter 4 Let's Play "Normal" or "Not Normal"

1. "The Postpartum Period," Cleveland Clinic, updated February 27, 2024, https://my.clevelandclinic.org/health/articles/postpartum.

2. Kelly B. Jouris et al., "The Effect of Omega-3 Fatty Acid Supplementation on the Inflammatory Response to Eccentric Strength Exercise," *Journal of Sports Science & Medicine* 10, no. 3 (2011): 432–38, https://pmc.ncbi.nlm.nih.gov/articles/PMC3737804/.

3. Cecilia M. Shing et al., "Acute Protease Supplementation Effects on Muscle Damage and Recovery Across Consecutive Days of Cycle Racing," *European Journal of Sport Science* 16, no. 2 (2016): 206–12, https://pubmed.ncbi.nlm.nih.gov/25604346/.

4. "Postpartum Hair Loss," Johns Hopkins Medicine, updated May 5, 2025, https://www.hopkinsmedicine.org/health/wellness-and-prevention/postpartum-hair-loss.

5. Robert S. English Jr. and James M. Barazesh, "Self-Assessments of Standardized Scalp Massages for Androgenic Alopecia: Survey Results," *Dermatology and Therapy* 9, no. 1 (2019): 167–78, https://doi.org/10.1007/s13555-019-0281-6.

6. Heather A. Hausenblas et al., "Magnesium-L-Threonate Improves Sleep Quality and Daytime Functioning in Adults with Self-Reported Sleep Problems: A Randomized Controlled Trial," *Sleep Medicine X* 8 (2024): 100121, https://pubmed.ncbi.nlm.nih.gov/39252819/.

7. Iulia O. Pfingstgraf et al., "Protective Effects of *Taraxacum officinale* L. (Dandelion) Root Extract in Experimental Acute on Chronic Liver Failure," *Antioxidants (Basel)* 10, no. 4 (2021): 504, https://pubmed.ncbi.nlm.nih.gov/33804908/.

8. Octavio Daniel Reyes-Hernández et al., "3,3'-Diindolylmethane and Indole-3-Carbinol: Potential Therapeutic Molecules for Cancer Chemoprevention and Treatment via Regulating Cellular Signaling Pathways," *Cancer Cell International* 23 (2023): 180, https://pmc.ncbi.nlm.nih.gov/articles/PMC10464192/.

9. Cynthia A. Thomson et al., "Chemopreventive Properties of 3,3'-Diindolylmethane in Breast Cancer: Evidence from Experimental and Human Studies," *Nutrition Reviews* 74, no. 7 (2016): 432–43, https://pmc.ncbi.nlm.nih.gov/articles/PMC5059820/.

10. "Evening Primrose," *Drugs and Lactation Database (LactMed®)*, May 17, 2021, https://www.ncbi.nlm.nih.gov/books/NBK501894/.

11. Jack H. Kessler, "The Effect of Supraphysiologic Levels of Iodine on Patients with Cyclic Mastalgia," *The Breast Journal* 10, no. 4 (2004): 328–36, https://pubmed.ncbi.nlm.nih.gov/15239792/.

12. R. Muggli, "Systemic Evening Primrose Oil Improves the Biophysical Skin Parameters of Healthy Adults," *International Journal of Cosmetic Science* 27, no. 4 (2005): 243–49, https://pubmed.ncbi.nlm.nih.gov/18492193/.

13. Moa Schalin-Karrila et al., "Evening Primrose Oil in the Treatment of Atopic Eczema: Effect on Clinical Status, Plasma Phospholipid Fatty Acids and Circulating Blood Prostaglandins," *British Journal of Dermatology* 117, no. 1 (1987): 11–19, https://onlinelibrary.wiley.com/doi/abs/10.1111/j.1365-2133.1987.tb04085.x.

14. See https://www.ewg.org/skindeep/.

15. Reyes-Hernández, "3,3'-Diindolylmethane and Indole-3-Carbinol," 180.

16. Elena Ugazio et al., "Ozonated Oils as Antimicrobial Systems in Topical Applications: Their Characterization, Current Applications, and Advances in Improved Delivery Techniques," *Molecules* 25, no. 2 (2020): 334, https://pmc.ncbi.nlm.nih.gov/articles/PMC7024311/.

17. H. O. Meissner et al., "Hormone-Balancing Effect of Pre-Gelatinized Organic Maca (Lepidium Peruvianum Chacon): (II) Physiological and Symptomatic Responses of Early-Postmenopausal Women to Standardized Doses of Maca in Double Blind, Randomized, Placebo-Controlled, Multi-Centre Clinical Study," *International Journal of Biomedical Science* 2, no. 4 (2006): 360–74, https://pmc.ncbi.nlm.nih.gov/articles/PMC3614647.

18. "Maca," E-Lactation, September 12, 2015, https://www.e-lactation.com/en/maca-pr/.

19. Keng-Liang Wu et al., "Effects of Ginger on Gastric Emptying and Motility in Healthy Humans," *European Journal of Gastroenterology & Hepatology* 20, no. 5 (2008): 436–40, https://pubmed.ncbi.nlm.nih.gov/18403946/.

20. Ping-Tao Tseng et al., "High Dosage Omega-3 Fatty Acids Outperform Existing Pharmacological Options for Migraine Prophylaxis: A Network Meta-Analysis," *Advances in Nutrition* 15, no. 2 (2024): 100163, https://pmc.ncbi.nlm.nih.gov/articles/PMC10808921/.

21. Sheyda Rezaie et al., "Effects of Curcumin Supplementation on Clinical Features and Inflammation in Migraine Patients: A Double-Blind Controlled, Placebo Randomized Clinical Trial," *International Journal of Preventive Medicine* 12 (December 1, 2021): 161, https://pmc.ncbi.nlm.nih.gov/articles/PMC8724631/.

Chapter 5 Nutritional Deficiencies

1. Thomas Ems et al., "Biochemistry, Iron Absorption," in *StatPearls* (StatPearls Publishing, 2025), https://www.ncbi.nlm.nih.gov/books/NBK448204/.

2. "Vitamin B_{12}—Health Professional Fact Sheet," National Institutes of Health, Office of Dietary Supplements, updated July 2, 2025, https://ods.od.nih.gov/factsheets/VitaminB12-HealthProfessional/.

3. "Medications Known to Decrease Vitamin B_{12} Levels," Evidence-Based Medicine Consult, updated October 2015, https://www.ebmconsult.com/articles/vitamin-b12-medication-interactions-lower-levels.

4. "Vitamin B_{12}," National Institutes of Health, Office of Dietary Supplements, https://ods.od.nih.gov/factsheets/VitaminB12-HealthProfessional/.

5. Lorena Carboni, "Active Folate Versus Folic Acid: The Role of 5-MTHF (Methylfolate) in Human Health," *Integrative Medicine* 21, no. 3 (2022): 36–41, https://www.ncbi.nlm.nih.gov/pmc/articles/PMC9380836/.

6. "Vitamin B_{12}," National Institutes of Health, Office of Dietary Supplements, https://ods.od.nih.gov/factsheets/VitaminB12-HealthProfessional/.

7. "Zinc: Fact Sheet for Health Professionals," National Institutes of Health, Office of Dietary Supplements, updated January 6, 2026, https://ods.od.nih.gov/factsheets/Zinc-HealthProfessional/.

8. Ambooken Betsy et al., "Zinc Deficiency Associated with Hypothyroidism: An Overlooked Cause of Severe Alopecia," *International Journal of Trichology* 5, no. 1 (2013): 40, https://doi.org/10.4103/0974-7753.114714.

9. Ambooken et al., "Zinc Deficiency Associated with Hypothyroidism."

10. Marzenna Nasiadek et al., "The Role of Zinc in Selected Female Reproductive System Disorders," *Nutrients* 12, no. 8 (2020): 2464, https://doi.org/10.3390/nu12082464.

11. Nancy F. Krebs, "Zinc Supplementation During Lactation," *American Journal of Clinical Nutrition* 68 (1998): 509S–12S, https://ajcn.nutrition.org/article/S0002-9165(23)00634-2/fulltext.

12. "Zinc," National Institutes of Health, Office of Dietary Supplements, https://ods.od.nih.gov/factsheets/Zinc-Consumer/.

13. B. Lönnerdal, "Dietary Factors Influencing Zinc Absorption," *Journal of Nutrition* 130 (May 2000): 1378S–83S, https://pubmed.ncbi.nlm.nih.gov/10801947/.

14. David R. Williams and Chiquita Collins, "US Socioeconomic and Racial Differences in Health: Patterns and Explanations," *Annual Review of Sociology* 21 (August 1995): 349–86, https://doi.org/10.1146/annurev.so.21.080195.002025.

15. "Zinc," National Institutes of Health, Office of Dietary Supplements, https://ods.od.nih.gov/factsheets/Zinc-HealthProfessional/.

16. Martin A. Kriegel et al., "Does Vitamin D Affect Risk of Developing Autoimmune Disease?" *Seminars in Arthritis and Rheumatism* 40, no. 6 (2011): 512–31, https://doi.org/10.1016/j.semarthrit.2010.07.009.

17. Sadia Kazi et al., "Effects of Vitamin D Supplementation on Muscle Function in Graves' Disease Patients," *Pakistan Journal of Medicine and Dentistry* 13, no. 4 (October 2024): 133–40.

18. Ippolita Valentina Di Molfetta et al., "Vitamin D and Its Role on the Fatigue Mitigation: A Narrative Review," *Nutrients* 16, no. 2 (2024): 221, https://doi.org/10.3390/nu16020221.

19. Sadia Sultan et al., "Low Vitamin D and Its Association with Cognitive Impairment and Dementia," *Journal of Aging Research* (April 30, 2020), https://doi.org/10.1155/2020/6097820.

20. Alessandro Cuomo et al., "Depression and Vitamin D Deficiency: Causality, Assessment, and Clinical Practice Implications," *Neuropsychiatry* 7, no. 5 (2017): 606–14, https://doi.org/10.4172/Neuropsychiatry.1000255.

21. Emad A. S. Al-Dujaili et al., "Effect of Vitamin D Supplementation on Cardiovascular Disease Risk Factors and Exercise Performance in Healthy Participants: A Randomized Placebo-Controlled Preliminary Study," *Therapeutic Advances in Endocrinology and Metabolism* 7, no. 4 (2016): 153–65, https://doi.org/10.1177/2042018816653357.

22. Krati Chauhan et al., "Vitamin D," in *StatPearls* (StatPearls Publishing, 2023), https://www.ncbi.nlm.nih.gov/books/NBK441912/.

23. Daniel D. Bikle, "Extraskeletal Actions of Vitamin D," *Annals of the New York Academy of Sciences* 1376, no. 1 (2016): 29–52, https://doi.org/10.1111/nyas.13219.

24. Sayed Esmaeil Mousavi et al., "Air Pollution, Environmental Chemicals, and Smoking May Trigger Vitamin D Deficiency: Evidence and

Potential Mechanisms," *Environment International* 122 (January 2019): 67–90, https://doi.org/10.1016/j.envint.2018.11.052.

25. Rebecca E. S. Anglin et al., "Vitamin D Deficiency and Depression in Adults: Systematic Review and Meta-Analysis," *British Journal of Psychiatry* 202 (2013): 100–7, https://pubmed.ncbi.nlm.nih.gov/23377209/.

26. Jasleen Kaur et al., "Vitamin D Deficiency," in *StatPearls* (StatPearls Publishing, 2025), https://www.ncbi.nlm.nih.gov/books/NBK532266/.

27. William Grant et al., "Vitamin D: Evidence-Based Health Benefits and Recommendations for Population Guidelines," *Nutrients* 17, no. 2 (2025): 277, https://doi.org/10.3390/nu17020277.

28. Esmail Mohammad Alayed Albarri et al., "Effectiveness of Vitamin D_2 Compared with Vitamin D_3 Replacement Therapy in a Primary Healthcare Setting: A Retrospective Cohort Study," *Qatar Medical Journal* 2022, no. 3 (2022): 29, https://doi.org/10.5339/qmj.2022.35.

29. Adriana J. van Ballegooijen et al., "The Synergistic Interplay Between Vitamins D and K for Bone and Cardiovascular Health: A Narrative Review," *International Journal of Endocrinology* (September 12, 2017), https://doi.org/10.1155/2017/7454376.

30. Janusz W. Krzyścin et al., "Optimal Vitamin D3 Daily Intake of 2000 IU Inferred from Modeled Solar Exposure of Ancestral Humans in Northern Tanzania," *Journal of Photochemistry and Photobiology B: Biology* 159 (June 2016): 101–5, https://doi.org/10.1016/j.jphotobiol.2016.03.029.

31. Debora Cutuli et al., "N-3 Polyunsaturated Fatty Acids Supplementation Enhances Hippocampal Functionality in Aged Mice," *Frontiers in Aging Neuroscience* 6 (August 25, 2014), https://doi.org/10.3389/fnagi.2014.00220.

32. Ricordi Poggioli et al., "Modulation of Inflammation and Immunity by Omega-3 Fatty Acids: A Possible Role for Prevention and to Halt Disease Progression in Autoimmune, Viral, and Age-Related Disorders," *European Review for Medical and Pharmacological Sciences* 27, no. 15 (2023): 7380–400, https://doi.org/10.26355/eurrev_202308_33310.

33. Lange Guo et al., "Association Between Polyunsaturated Fatty Acid Intake and Estradiol Levels Among US Women," *Frontiers in Nutrition* 11 (November 2024), https://doi.org/10.3389/fnut.2024.1500705.

34. Annelise A. Madison et al., "Omega-3 Supplementation and Stress Reactivity of Cellular Aging Biomarkers: An Ancillary Substudy of a Randomized, Controlled Trial in Midlife Adults," *Molecular Psychiatry* 26, no. 7 (2021): 3034–42, https://doi.org/10.1038/s41380-021-01077-2.

35. Yuhua Liao et al., "Efficacy of Omega-3 PUFAs in Depression: A Meta-Analysis," *Translational Psychiatry* 9 (2019): 465, https://doi.org/10.1038/s41398-021-01582-6.

36. Jeanette Y. Ziegenfuss et al., "Behaviors, Beliefs, and Recommendations to Optimize Promotion of Safe Fish Consumption Before and During Pregnancy: A Physician Survey," *Journal of Primary Care & Community Health* 13 (2022), https://doi.org/10.1177/21501319221126980.

37. "Is It Okay to Eat Fish Every Day?" Harvard T. H. Chan School of Public Health News, updated November 21, 2024, https://hsph.harvard.edu/news/is-it-okay-to-eat-fish-every-day/.

Chapter 6 Thyroid Disorders

1. Karen Carlson and Beverly A. Mikes, "Postpartum Thyroiditis," in *StatPearls* (StatPearls Publishing, 2025), https://www.ncbi.nlm.nih.gov/books/NBK557646/.

2. Karsten Müssig et al., "Thyroid Peroxidase Antibody Positivity Is Associated with Symptomatic Distress in Patients with Hashimoto's Thyroiditis," *Brain, Behavior, and Immunity* 26, no. 4 (2012): 559–63, https://doi.org/10.1016/j.bbi.2012.01.006.

3. Alex Stagnaro-Green, "Approach to the Patient with Postpartum Thyroiditis," *Journal of Clinical Endocrinology & Metabolism* 97, no. 2 (2012): 334–42, https://doi.org/10.1210/jc.2011-2576.

4. S. Mariotti et al., "Antithyroid Peroxidase Autoantibodies in Thyroid Diseases," *Journal of Clinical Endocrinology & Metabolism* 71, no. 3 (1990): 661–69, https://doi.org/10.1210/jcem-71-3-661.

5. Frederick W. Miller, "The Increasing Prevalence of Autoimmunity and Autoimmune Diseases: An Urgent Call to Action for Improved Understanding, Diagnosis, Treatment, and Prevention," *Current Opinion in Immunology* 80 (February 2023): 102266, https://doi.org/10.1016/j.coi.2022.102266.

6. Yuji Shimizu et al., "The Association Between Anti-Thyroid Peroxidase Antibody and Thyroid Stimulating Hormone: A Cross-Sectional Study," *Scientific Reports* 13, no. 1 (2023): 14358, https://doi.org/10.1038/s41598-023-40275-6.

7. Carlson and Mikes, "Postpartum Thyroiditis."

8. Kimberly Dorris, "American Thyroid Association Task Force Updates Guidelines on Thyroid Disease and Pregnancy," *Clinical Thyroidology for the Public* 10, no. 5 (2017): 3–7, https://www.thyroid.org/patient-thyroid-information/ct-for-patients/may-2017/vol-10-issue-5-p-3-7/.

9. Meghna Shah et al., "A Tale of Two Therapies: A Comparison of Armour Thyroid and Levothyroxine," *Journal of the Endocrine Society* 5, supplement 1 (2021), https://doi.org/10.1210/jendso/bvab048.1678.

10. Yong-Sheng Wang et al., "The Effects of Selenium Supplementation in the Treatment of Autoimmune Thyroiditis: An Overview of Systematic

Reviews," *Nutrients* 15, no. 14 (2023): 3194, https://doi.org/10.3390/nu15143194.

11. Elias E. Mazokopakis et al., "Effects of 12 Months Treatment with L-Selenomethionine on Serum Anti-TPO Levels in Patients with Hashimoto's Thyroiditis," *Thyroid* 17, no. 7 (2007): 609–12, https://doi.org/10.1089/thy.2007.0040.

12. Nadiya Pasyechko and Veronika Kulchinska, "Myo-Inositol Supplementation in Autoimmune Thyroiditis and Subclinical Hypothyroidism on the Background of Vitamin D Deficiency," *Endocrine Abstracts* 81 (2022): EP1068, https://doi.org/10.1530/endoabs.81.EP1068.

13. Maurizio Nordio and Sabrina Basciani, "Treatment with Myo-Inositol and Selenium Ensures Euthyroidism in Patients with Autoimmune Thyroiditis," *International Journal of Endocrinology* (2017), https://doi.org/10.1155/2017/2549491.

14. Denise K. Patten et al., "The Safety and Efficacy of Low-Dose Naltrexone in the Management of Chronic Pain and Inflammation in Multiple Sclerosis, Fibromyalgia, Crohn's Disease, and Other Chronic Pain Disorders," *Pharmacotherapy* 38, no. 3 (2018): 382–89, https://doi.org/10.1002/phar.2086.

15. Zijian Li et al., "Low-Dose Naltrexone (LDN): A Promising Treatment in Immune-Related Diseases and Cancer Therapy," *International Immunopharmacology* 61 (August 2018): 178–84, https://doi.org/10.1016/j.intimp.2018.05.020.

16. Maria E. Street et al., "The Impact of Environmental Factors and Contaminants on Thyroid Function and Disease from Fetal to Adult Life: Current Evidence and Future Directions," *Frontiers in Endocrinology* 15 (2024): 1429884, https://doi.org/10.3389/fendo.2024.1429884.

17. Tommaso Piticchio et al., "Effect of Gluten-Free Diet on Autoimmune Thyroiditis Progression in Patients with No Symptoms or Histology of Celiac Disease: A Meta-Analysis," *Frontiers in Endocrinology* 14 (July 24, 2023): 1200372, https://doi.org/10.3389/fendo.2023.1200372.

18. Jovana Knezevic et al., "Thyroid-Gut-Axis: How Does the Microbiota Influence Thyroid Function?" *Nutrients* 12, no. 6 (2020), https://doi.org/10.3390/nu12061769.

19. Xuefang Liu et al., "Significance of Monitoring the Levels of Thyroid Hormone Antibodies and Glucose and Lipid Metabolism Antibodies in Patients Suffering from Type 2 Diabetes," *Open Medicine* 18, no. 1 (2023), https://doi.org/10.1515/med-2023-0876.

20. Erik Stokstad, "Perchlorate Impacts Thyroid at Low Doses," *Science*, October 6, 2006, https://www.science.org/content/article/perchlorate-impacts-thyroid-low-doses.

21. Mary E. Turyk et al., "Relationships of Thyroid Hormones with Polychlorinated Biphenyls, Dioxins, Furans, and DDE in Adults," *Environmental Health Perspectives* 115, no. 8 (2007): 1197–203, https://pmc.ncbi.nlm.nih.gov/articles/PMC1940071/.

22. R. Thomas Zoeller, "Environmental Chemicals Impacting the Thyroid: Targets and Consequences," *Thyroid* 17, no. 9 (2007): 811–17, https://doi.org/10.1089/thy.2007.0107.

23. Rakesh Balachandar et al., "Association Between Blood Lead Levels and Thyroid Function: An Updated Systematic Review and Meta-Analysis," *Indian Journal of Clinical Biochemistry* 38, no. 4 (2023): 426–36, https://doi.org/10.1007/s12291-023-01113-8.

24. Kevin M. Rice et al., "Environmental Mercury and Its Toxic Effects," *Journal of Preventive Medicine and Public Health* 47, no. 2 (2014): 74–83, https://doi.org/10.3961/jpmph.2014.47.2.74.

25. "Hyperthyroidism (Overactive Thyroid)," Mayo Clinic, updated November 30, 2022, https://www.mayoclinic.org/diseases-conditions/hyperthyroidism/symptoms-causes/syc-20373659.

26. Salvatore Benvenga et al., "Nutraceutical Supplements in the Thyroid Setting: Health Benefits Beyond Basic Nutrition," *Nutrients* 11, no. 9 (2019): 2214, https://doi.org/10.3390/nu11092214.

27. Daniel Kaplan and Chrysoula Dosiou, "Two Cases of Graves' Hyperthyroidism Treated with Homeopathic Remedies Containing Herbal Extracts from *Lycopus spp*. and *Melissa officinalis*," *Journal of the Endocrine Society* 5 (May 2021): A971, https://doi.org/10.1210/jendso/bvab048.1984.

28. Zhuoshi Yang et al., "Effect of Traditional Chinese Medicine on Graves' Disease: A Network Meta-Analysis," *Frontiers in Pharmacology* 15 (August 22, 2024): article 1411459, https://doi.org/10.3389/fphar.2024.1411459.

29. Jessica Farebrother et al., "Excess Iodine Intake: Sources, Assessment, and Effects on Thyroid Function," *Annals of the New York Academy of Sciences* 1446, no. 1 (2019): 44–65, https://doi.org/10.1111/nyas.14041.

30. Fereidoun Azizi et al., "Increased Remission Rates After Long-Term Methimazole Therapy in Patients with Graves' Disease: Results of a Randomized Clinical Trial," *Thyroid* 29, no. 9 (2019): 1192–200, https://doi.org/10.1089/thy.2019.0180.

31. Stagnaro-Green, "Approach to the Patient," 334–42.

32. Stagnaro-Green, "Approach to the Patient," 334–42.

33. Tetsuya Mizokami et al., "Stress and Thyroid Autoimmunity," *Thyroid* 14, no. 12 (2004): 1047–55, https://doi.org/10.1089/thy.2004.14.1047.

Chapter 7 Autoimmunity

1. Syreen Goulmamine et al., "Autoimmune Health Crisis: An Inclusive Approach to Addressing Disparities in Women in the United States," *International Journal of Environmental Research and Public Health* 21, no. 10 (2024): 1339, https://doi.org/10.3390/ijerph21101339.

2. Ali S. Khashan et al., "Pregnancy and the Risk of Autoimmune Disease," *PLoS One* 6, no. 5 (2011): e19658, https://doi.org/10.1371/journal.pone.0019658.

3. Natalie V. Scime et al., "Pregnancy Complications and New-Onset Maternal Autoimmune Disease," *International Journal of Epidemiology* 53, no. 5 (2024), https://doi.org/10.1093/ije/dyae115.

4. Massimo Tonacchera et al., "Relative Potencies and Additivity of Perchlorate, Thiocyanate, Nitrate, and Iodide on the Inhibition of Radioactive Iodide Uptake by the Human Sodium Iodide Symporter," *Thyroid* 14, no. 12 (December 2004): 1012–19, https://doi.org/10.1089/thy.2004.14.1012.

5. Goulmamine et al., "Autoimmune Health Crisis."

6. Jane Henderson et al., "Factors Associated with Maternal Postpartum Fatigue: An Observational Study," *BMJ Open* 9, no. 7 (2019): e025927, https://doi.org/10.1136/bmjopen-2018-025927.

7. David Richter et al., "Long-Term Effects of Pregnancy and Childbirth on Sleep Satisfaction and Duration of First-Time and Experienced Mothers and Fathers," *Sleep* 42, no. 4 (2019): zsz015, https://doi.org/10.1093/sleep/zsz015.

8. S. Gizlenti and T. R. Ekmekci, "The Changes in the Hair Cycle During Gestation and the Post-Partum Period," *Journal of the European Academy of Dermatology and Venereology* 28, no. 7 (2014): 878–81, https://doi.org/10.1111/jdv.12188.

9. Madison J. Anzelc and Mark A. Bechtel, "Considerations for Cutaneous Physiologic Changes of Pregnancy That Fail to Resolve Postpartum," *International Journal of Dermatology* 62, no. 2 (2023): 190–96, https://doi.org/10.1111/ijd.16105.

10. Doris Wilborn et al., "Relationships Between Skin Structure and Skin Function of Pregnant Women and Their Infants: A Prospective Cohort Study," *Skin Pharmacology and Physiology* 38, no. 4 (2025), https://doi.org/10.1159/000546770.

11. Anne Marie Gausel et al., "Subjective Recovery from Pregnancy-Related Pelvic Girdle Pain the First 6 Weeks after Delivery: A Prospective Longitudinal Cohort Study," *European Spine Journal* 29, no. 3 (2020): 556–63, https://doi.org/10.1007/s00586-020-06288-9.

12. Satish S. C. Rao et al., "Constipation, Hemorrhoids, and Anorectal Disorders in Pregnancy," *American Journal of Gastroenterology* 117, no. 10S (2022): 16–25, https://doi.org/10.14309/ajg.0000000000001962.

13. M. Pikwer et al., "Breast Feeding, but Not Use of Oral Contraceptives, Is Associated with a Reduced Risk of Rheumatoid Arthritis," *Annals of the Rheumatic Diseases* 68, no. 4 (2009): 526–30, https://doi.org/10.1136/ard.2007.084707.

14. Sung-Woo Kim et al., "Association of Breastfeeding with Thyroid Function and Autoimmunity in Postmenopausal Women," *Endocrine* 71, no. 1 (2021): 130–38, https://doi.org/10.1007/s12020-020-02385-3.

15. Sara Collorone et al., "The Protective Role of Breastfeeding in Multiple Sclerosis: Latest Evidence and Practical Considerations," *Frontiers in Neurology* 13 (2023): 1090133, https://doi.org/10.3389/fneur.2022.1090133.

16. Anna Julkunen et al., "Autoimmune Diseases and Oral Health: 30-Year Follow-Up of a Swedish Cohort," *Dentistry Journal* 6, no. 1 (2018): 1, https://doi.org/10.3390/dj6010001.

17. Blaine Caslin et al., "Alcohol as Friend or Foe in Autoimmune Diseases: A Role for Gut Microbiome?" *Gut Microbes* 13, no. 1 (2021): 1916278, https://doi.org/10.1080/19490976.2021.1916278.

18. Sakinah Othman et al., "Postpartum Thyroiditis: An Organ-Specific Syndrome Which Is Not Associated with a Postpartum Polyclonal B-Cell Activation," *Autoimmunity* 13, no. 4 (1995): 33–36, https://doi.org/10.3109/08916939209112343.

19. April Barnado et al., "Identifying Antinuclear Antibody Positive Individuals at Risk for Developing Systemic Autoimmune Disease: Development and Validation of a Real-Time Risk Model," *Frontiers in Immunology* 15 (March 20, 2024), https://doi.org/10.3389/fimmu.2024.1384229.

20. Jessica A. Reese et al., "Platelet Counts During Pregnancy," *New England Journal of Medicine* 379, no. 1 (2018): 24–34, https://doi.org/10.1056/NEJMoa1802897.

21. K. Mertens et al., "Postpartum C-Reactive Protein: A Limited Value to Detect Infection or Inflammation," *Facts, Views & Vision in ObGyn* 11, no. 3 (2019): 243–50, https://www.ncbi.nlm.nih.gov/pmc/articles/PMC7020948/.

22. Megha Singh et al., "Pregnancy Complications and Autoimmune Diseases in Women: Systematic Review and Meta-Analysis," *BMC Medicine* 22, no. 1 (2024): 339, https://doi.org/10.1186/s12916-024-03550-5.

23. Pamela M. Williams et al., "Celiac Disease: Common Questions and Answers," *American Family Physician* 106, no. 1 (2022): 36–43, https://pubmed.ncbi.nlm.nih.gov/35839368/.

24. Steffen Husby et al., "AGA Clinical Practice Update on Diagnosis and Monitoring of Celiac Disease: Changing Utility of Serology and

Histologic Measures: Expert Review," *Gastroenterology* 156, no. 4 (2019): 885–89, https://doi.org/10.1053/j.gastro.2018.12.010.

25. Deepti Upadhyay et al., "Can Arginine, Glutamate and Glutamine Serve as Surrogates of Intestinal Mucosal Healing in the Patients with Celiac Disease Following Gluten-Free Diet? An NMR-Based Metabolomics Study," *Magnetic Resonance Imaging* 121 (September 2025): article 110421, https://doi.org/10.1016/j.mri.2025.110421.

26. Caroline L. Seiler et al., "Probiotics for Celiac Disease: A Systematic Review and Meta-Analysis of Randomized Controlled Trials," *American Journal of Gastroenterology* 115, no. 10 (2020): 1584–95, https://doi.org/10.14309/ajg.0000000000000749.

27. Guoxian Wei et al., "Gluten Degrading Enzymes for Treatment of Celiac Disease," *Nutrients* 12, no. 7 (2020): 2095, https://doi.org/10.3390/nu12072095.

28. Joseph D. Feuerstein et al., "American Gastroenterological Association Institute Clinical Guideline on the Management of Moderate to Severe Ulcerative Colitis," *Gastroenterology* 158, no. 5 (2020): 1450–61, https://doi.org/10.1053/j.gastro.2020.01.006.

29. Gary R. Lichtenstein et al., "ACG Clinical Guideline: Management of Crohn's Disease in Adults," *American Journal of Gastroenterology* 113, no. 4 (2018): 481–517, https://doi.org/10.1038/ajg.2018.27.

30. Georgios Vakadaris et al., "The Role of Probiotics in Inducing and Maintaining Remission in Crohn's Disease and Ulcerative Colitis: A Systematic Review of the Literature," *Biomedicines* 11, no. 2 (2023): 494, https://doi.org/10.3390/biomedicines11020494.

31. Adrian Goldiş et al., "Clinical Efficacy of Sodium Butyrate in Managing Pediatric Inflammatory Bowel Disease," *Life* 15, no. 6 (2025): 902, https://doi.org/10.3390/life15060902.

32. Rinkalben Kakdiya et al., "Indigo Naturalis (Qing Dai) for Inflammatory Bowel Disease: A Systematic Review and Meta-Analysis," *Clinics and Research in Hepatology and Gastroenterology* 48, no. 1 (2024): 102250, https://doi.org/10.1016/j.clinre.2023.102250.

33. Camila dos Santos Leite et al., "The Anti-Inflammatory Properties of Licorice (*Glycyrrhiza glabra*)-Derived Compounds in Intestinal Disorders," *International Journal of Molecular Sciences* 23, no. 8 (2022): 4121, https://doi.org/10.3390/ijms23084121.

34. Saeid Mohseni et al., "Curcumin for the Clinical Treatment of Inflammatory Bowel Diseases: A Systematic Review and Meta-Analysis of Placebo-Controlled Randomized Clinical Trials," *Frontiers in Nutrition* 12 (March 24, 2025): 1494351, https://doi.org/10.3389/fnut.2025.1494351.

35. Emily Peterson et al., "Rheumatoid Arthritis: Diagnosis and Management for the Family Physician," *American Family Physician*, 110, no. 5

(2024): 515–26, https://www.aafp.org/pubs/afp/issues/2024/1100/rheuma toid-arthritis.html.

36. "Management of Rheumatoid Arthritis: Update From ACR," *American Family Physician* 106, no. 3 (2022): 340–42, https://www.aafp.org/pubs/afp /issues/2022/0900/practice-guidelines-rheumatoid-arthritis.html.

37. Caroline H. Siegel and Lisa R. Sammaritano, "Systemic Lupus Erythematosus," *JAMA* 331, no. 17 (2024): 1480–91, https://doi.org/10.1001 /jama.2024.2315.

38. Sandy Nasr and Andras Perl, "Principles Behind SLE Treatment with *N*-Acetylcysteine," *Immunometabolism* 4, no. 4 (2022): e00010, https://doi .org/10.1097/IN9.0000000000000010.

39. Jörg Leipner et al., "Therapy with Proteolytic Enzymes in Rheumatic Disorders," *BioDrugs* 15, no. 12 (2001): 779–89, https://doi.org/10.2165 /00063030-200115120-00001.

40. Niriksha Ravi et al., "The Key Role of Glutathione Compared to Curcumin in the Management of Systemic Lupus Erythematosus: A Systematic Review," *Cureus* 14, no. 11 (2022): e31324, https://doi.org/10.7759 /cureus.31324.

41. Marisa P. McGinley et al., "Diagnosis and Treatment of Multiple Sclerosis: A Review," *JAMA* 325, no. 8 (2021): 765–79, https://doi.org/10 .1001/jama.2020.26858.

42. Panayiotis Aristotelous et al., "The Effects of Specific Omega-3 and Omega-6 Polyunsaturated Fatty Acids and Antioxidant Vitamins on Gait and Functional Capacity Parameters in Patients with Relapsing-Remitting Multiple Sclerosis," *Nutrients* 13, no. 10 (2021): 3661, https://doi.org/10 .3390/nu13103661.

43. Ethel Ciampi et al., "Efficacy of Andrographolide in Not Active Progressive Multiple Sclerosis: A Prospective Exploratory Double-Blind, Parallel-Group, Randomized, Placebo-Controlled Trial," *BMC Neurology* 20 (2020): 173, https://doi.org/10.1186/s12883-020-01745-w.

44. Alireza Shadab et al., "Exploring the Immune-Modulating Properties of Boswellic Acid in Experimental Autoimmune Encephalomyelitis," *APMIS* 132, no. 6 (2024): 452–64, https://doi.org/10.1111/apm.13406.

45. Thorsten Rudroff and Jacob Sosnoff, "Cannabidiol to Improve Mobility in People with Multiple Sclerosis," *Frontiers in Neurology* 9 (2018): 183, https://doi.org/10.3389/fneur.2018.00183.

46. April W. Armstrong et al., "Pathophysiology, Clinical Presentation, and Treatment of Psoriasis: A Review," *JAMA* 323, no. 19 (2020): 1945–60, https://doi.org/10.1001/jama.2020.4006.

47. Chunxiao Wang et al., "Evidence and Potential Mechanism of Action of Indigo Naturalis and Its Active Components in the Treatment of

Psoriasis," *Annals of Medicine* 56, no. 1 (2024): 2329261, https://doi.org/10.1080/07853890.2024.2329261.

48. Monica Janeczek et al., "Review of the Efficacy and Safety of Topical *Mahonia aquifolium* for the Treatment of Psoriasis and Atopic Dermatitis," *Journal of Clinical and Aesthetic Dermatology* 11, no. 12 (2018): 42–47.

49. Shuo Zhang et al., "Efficacy and Safety of Curcumin in Psoriasis: Preclinical and Clinical Evidence and Possible Mechanisms," *Frontiers in Pharmacology* 13 (2022): 903160, https://doi.org/10.3389/fphar.2022.903160.

50. Mihaela Cristina Buhaş et al., "Transforming Psoriasis Care: Probiotics and Prebiotics as Novel Therapeutic Approaches," *International Journal of Molecular Sciences* 24, no. 13 (2023): 11225, https://doi.org/10.3390/ijms241311225.

Chapter 8 Adrenal Dysfunction

1. Caroline Jung et al., "A Longitudinal Study of Plasma and Urinary Cortisol in Pregnancy and Postpartum," *The Journal of Clinical Endocrinology & Metabolism* 96, no. 5 (2011): 1533–40, https://doi.org/10.1210/jc.2010-2395.

2. G. Mastorakos and I. Ilias, "Maternal Hypothalamic-Pituitary-Adrenal Axis in Pregnancy and the Postpartum Period: Postpartum-Related Disorders," *Annals of the New York Academy of Sciences* 900 (2000): 95–106, https://doi.org/10.1111/j.1749-6632.2000.tb06220.x.

3. David S. Goldstein, "Adrenal Responses to Stress," *Cellular and Molecular Neurobiology* 30, no. 8 (2010): 1433–40, https://doi.org/10.1007/s10571-010-9606-9.

4. Vadim Tseilikman et al., "Role of Glucocorticoid- and Monoamine-Metabolizing Enzymes in Stress-Related Psychopathological Processes," *Stress* 23, no. 1 (2019): 1–12, https://doi.org/10.1080/10253890.2019.1641080.

5. Brianna Chu et al., "Physiology, Stress Reaction," in *StatPearls* (StatPearls Publishing, 2024), https://www.ncbi.nlm.nih.gov/books/NBK541120/.

6. "Common Patterns of Cortisol Imbalance," ZRT Laboratory, September 8, 2017, https://www.zrtlab.com/media/1488/pho-common-cortisol.pdf.

7. Chu, "Physiology, Stress Reaction."

8. "Common Patterns of Cortisol Imbalance," ZRT Laboratory.

9. J. Delarue et al., "Fish Oil Prevents the Adrenal Activation Elicited by Mental Stress in Healthy Men," *Diabetes & Metabolism* 29, no. 3 (2003): 289–95, https://doi.org/10.1016/s1262-3636(07)70039-3.

10. Narine Beglaryan et al., "Vitamin C Supplementation Alleviates Hypercortisolemia Caused by Chronic Stress," *Stress and Health* 40, no. 3 (2024): e3347, https://doi.org/10.1002/smi.3347.

11. Juliane Hellhammer et al., "A Soy-Based Phosphatidylserine/Phosphatidic Acid Complex (PAS) Normalizes the Stress Reactivity of Hypothalamus-Pituitary-Adrenal-Axis in Chronically Stressed Male Subjects: A Randomized, Placebo-Controlled Study," *Lipids in Health and Disease* 13 (July 31, 2014): 121, https://doi.org/10.1186/1476-511X-13-121.

12. Shawn M. Talbott et al., "Effect of *Magnolia officinalis* and *Phellodendron amurense* (Relora®) on Cortisol and Psychological Mood State in Moderately Stressed Subjects," *Journal of the International Society of Sports Nutrition* 10, no. 1 (2013): 37, https://doi.org/10.1186/1550-2783-10-37.

13. Matteo Della Porta et al., "Effects of *Withania somnifera* on Cortisol Levels in Stressed Human Subjects: A Systematic Review," *Nutrients* 15, no. 24 (2023): 5015, https://doi.org/10.3390/nu15245015.

14. Erik M. Olsson et al., "A Randomised, Double-Blind, Placebo-Controlled, Parallel-Group Study of the Standardised Extract SHR-5 of the Roots of *Rhodiola rosea* in the Treatment of Subjects with Stress-Related Fatigue," *Planta Medica* 75, no. 2 (2009): 105–12, https://doi.org/10.1055/s-0028-1088346.

15. Chiara Sabbadin et al., "Licorice: From Pseudohyperaldosteronism to Therapeutic Uses," *Frontiers in Endocrinology* 10 (July 18, 2019): 484, https://doi.org/10.3389/fendo.2019.00484.

16. Hannah M. Costello et al., "High Salt Intake Activates the Hypothalamic-Pituitary-Adrenal Axis, Amplifies the Stress Response, and Alters Tissue Glucocorticoid Exposure in Mice," *Cardiovascular Research* 119, no. 8 (2023): 1740–50, https://doi.org/10.1093/cvr/cvac160.

17. Agnieszka Pazderska and Simon H. S. Pearce, "Adrenal Insufficiency—Recognition and Management," *Clinical Medicine* 17, no. 3 (2017): 258–62, https://doi.org/10.7861/clinmedicine.17-3-258.

Chapter 9 Insulin Resistance

1. "Free Keyword Research Tool," Wordtracker, accessed March 9, 2026, https://www.wordtracker.com/.

2. Diana C. Soria-Contreras et al., "Weight Trajectories After Delivery Are Associated with Adiposity and Cardiometabolic Markers at 3 Years Postpartum Among Women in Project Viva," *Journal of Nutrition* 150, no. 7 (2020): 1889–98, https://doi.org/10.1093/jn/nxaa104.

3. Soria-Contreras et al., "Weight Trajectories After Delivery," 1889–98.

4. Heather L. Paladine et al., "Postpartum Care: An Approach to the Fourth Trimester," *American Family Physician* 100, no. 8 (2019): 485–91, https://www.aafp.org/pubs/afp/issues/2019/1015/p485.html.

5. Soria-Contreras et al., "Weight Trajectories After Delivery," 1889–98.

6. Mitsugu Shimobayashi et al., "Insulin Resistance Causes Inflammation in Adipose Tissue," *Journal of Clinical Investigation* 128, no. 4 (2018): 1538–50, https://doi.org/10.1172/JCI96139.

7. Philipp Mergenthaler et al., "Sugar for the Brain: The Role of Glucose in Physiological and Pathological Brain Function," *Trends in Neurosciences* 36, no. 10 (2013): 587–97, https://doi.org/10.1016/j.tins.2013.07.001.

8. Thomas M. Barber et al., "Mechanisms of Insulin Resistance at the Crossroad of Obesity with Associated Metabolic Abnormalities and Cognitive Dysfunction," *International Journal of Molecular Sciences* 22, no. 2 (2021): 546, https://doi.org/10.3390/ijms22020546.

9. Ana G. Gutiérrez García and Carlos M. Contreras, "Anxiety Constitutes an Early Sign of Acute Hypoglycemia," *Neuropsychobiology* 82, no. 1 (2023): 33–39, https://doi.org/10.1159/000528351.

10. Judith Gruber et al., "Impact of Insulin and Insulin Resistance on Brain Dopamine Signalling and Reward Processing—An Underexplored Mechanism in the Pathophysiology of Depression?" *Neuroscience & Biobehavioral Reviews* 149 (June 2023): 105179y, https://doi.org/10.1016/j.neubiorev.2023.105179.

11. Mona Ali et al., "The Potential Impact of Insulin Resistance and Metabolic Syndrome on Migraine Headache Characteristics," *BMC Neurology* 22, no. 1 (2022): 422, https://doi.org/10.1186/s12883-022-02966-x.

12. Vinay Maudar et al., "Hot Flashes and Fatigue Relieved by Metformin," *Endocrine Practice* 15, no. 1 (2009): 30–34, https://doi.org/10.4158/EP.15.1.30.

13. Magdalini Kreouzi et al., "Skin Microbiota: Mediator of Interactions Between Metabolic Disorders and Cutaneous Health and Disease," *Microorganisms* 13, no. 1 (2025): 161, https://doi.org/10.3390/microorganisms13010161.

14. Kristin A. McAuley et al., "Diagnosing Insulin Resistance in the General Population," *Diabetes Care* 24, no. 3 (2001): 460–64, https://doi.org/10.2337/diacare.24.3.460.

15. Asghar Ghasemi et al., "Cut-Off Points of Homeostasis Model Assessment of Insulin Resistance, Beta-Cell Function, and Fasting Serum Insulin to Identify Future Type 2 Diabetes: Tehran Lipid and Glucose Study," *Acta Diabetologica* 52, no. 5 (2015): 905–15, https://doi.org/10.1007/s00592-015-0730-3; Y. Gallois et al., "Distribution of Fasting Serum Insulin Measured by Enzyme Immunoassay in an Unselected Population of 4,032 Individuals: Reference Values According to Age and Sex. D.E.S.I.R. Study Group

(Données Épidémiologiques sur le Syndrome d'Insulino-Résistance)," *Diabetes & Metabolism* 22, no. 6 (1996): 427–31, https://pubmed.ncbi.nlm.nih.gov/8985651/.

16. Steven E. Stern et al., "Identification of Individuals with Insulin Resistance Using Routine Clinical Measurements," *Diabetes* 54, no. 2 (2005): 333–39, https://doi.org/10.2337/diabetes.54.2.333.

17. Juan F. Ascaso et al., "Insulin Resistance Quantification by Fasting Insulin Plasma Values and HOMA Index in a Non-Diabetic Population," *Medicina Clínica* 117, no. 14 (2001): 530–33, https://doi.org/10.1016/S0025-7753(01)72168-9.

18. Richard S. Surwit et al., "Stress and Diabetes Mellitus," *Diabetes Care* 15, no. 10 (1992): 1413–22, https://doi.org/10.2337/diacare.15.10.1413.

19. Carlos Lorenzo et al., "A1C between 5.7 and 6.4% as a Marker for Identifying Pre-Diabetes, Insulin Sensitivity and Secretion, and Cardiovascular Risk Factors: The Insulin Resistance Atherosclerosis Study (IRAS)," *Diabetes Care* 33, no. 9 (2010): 2104–9, https://doi.org/10.2337/dc10-0679.

20. James L. Rosenzweig et al., "Primary Prevention of ASCVD and T2DM in Patients at Metabolic Risk: An Endocrine Society Clinical Practice Guideline," *Journal of Clinical Endocrinology & Metabolism* 104, no. 9 (2019): 3939–85, https://doi.org/10.1210/jc.2019-01338.

21. Aditya K. Khetan and Sanjay Rajagopalan, "Prediabetes," *Canadian Journal of Cardiology* 34, no. 5 (2018): 615–23, https://doi.org/10.1016/j.cjca.2017.12.030.

22. Vibhu Parcha et al., "Insulin Resistance and Cardiometabolic Risk Profile Among Nondiabetic American Young Adults: Insights from NHANES," *Journal of Clinical Endocrinology & Metabolism* 107, no. 1 (2022): e25–e37, https://doi.org/10.1210/clinem/dgab645.

23. Marisol Cortez-Navarrete et al., "Role of Fenugreek, Cinnamon, *Curcuma longa*, Berberine and *Momordica charantia* in Type 2 Diabetes Mellitus Treatment: A Review," *Pharmaceuticals* 16, no. 4 (2023): 515, https://doi.org/10.3390/ph16040515.

24. Tahir Mehmood Khan et al., "Effectiveness of Fenugreek as a Galactagogue: A Network Meta-Analysis," *Phytotherapy Research* 32, no. 3 (2018): 402–12, https://doi.org/10.1002/ptr.5972.

25. Charmie Fong et al., "Efficacy and Safety of Nutrient Supplements for Glycaemic Control and Insulin Resistance in Type 2 Diabetes: An Umbrella Review and Hierarchical Evidence Synthesis," *Nutrients* 14, no. 11 (2022): 2295, https://doi.org/10.3390/nu14112295.

26. Chengcheng Zhang et al., "Meta-Analysis of Randomized Controlled Trials of the Effects of Probiotics on Type 2 Diabetes in Adults," *Clinical Nutrition* 41, no. 2 (2022): 365–73, https://doi.org/10.1016/j.clnu.2021.11.037.

27. Hui-Hui Guo et al., "Berberine Is a Potential Alternative for Metformin with Good Regulatory Effect on Lipids in Treating Metabolic Diseases," *Biomedicine & Pharmacotherapy* 163 (July 2023): 114754, https://doi.org/10.1016/j.biopha.2023.114754; Jun Yin et al., "Efficacy of Berberine in Patients with Type 2 Diabetes," *Metabolism* 57, no. 5 (2008): 712–17, https://doi.org/10.1016/j.metabol.2008.01.013; Haoran Wang et al., "Metformin and Berberine, Two Versatile Drugs in Treatment of Common Metabolic Diseases," *Oncotarget* 9, no. 11 (2017): 10135–46, https://doi.org/10.18632/oncotarget.20807.

Chapter 11 Depression, Anxiety, and Other Mental Health Concerns

1. Karen Carlson et al., "Perinatal Depression," in *StatPearls* (StatPearls Publishing, 2025), https://www.ncbi.nlm.nih.gov/books/NBK519070/.

2. Brenda L. Bauman, "Vital Signs: Postpartum Depressive Symptoms and Provider Discussions About Perinatal Depression—United States, 2018," *Morbidity and Mortality Weekly Report* 69, no. 19 (2020): 575–81, https://doi.org/10.15585/mmwr.mm6919a2.

3. Silvia Manso-Córdoba et al., "Factors Related to Seeking Help for Postpartum Depression: A Secondary Analysis of New York City PRAMS Data," *International Journal of Environmental Research and Public Health* 17, no. 24 (2020): 9328, https://doi.org/10.3390/ijerph17249328.

4. Nicole Vliegen et al., "The Course of Postpartum Depression: A Review of Longitudinal Studies," *Harvard Review of Psychiatry* 22, no. 1 (2014): 1–22, https://doi.org/10.1097/HRP.0000000000000013.

5. Nehaa Khadka et al., "Trends in Postpartum Depression by Race, Ethnicity, and Prepregnancy Body Mass Index," *JAMA Network Open* 7, no. 11 (2024): e2446486, https://doi.org/10.1001/jamanetworkopen.2024.46486.

6. Fanie Collardeau et al., "Prevalence and Course of Unwanted, Intrusive Thoughts of Infant-Related Harm," *Journal of Clinical Psychiatry* 85, no. 3 (2024): 23m15145, https://doi.org/10.4088/JCP.23m15145.

7. Yael I. Nillni et al., "Treatment of Depression, Anxiety, and Trauma-Related Disorders During the Perinatal Period: A Systematic Review," *Clinical Psychology Review* 66 (December 2018): 136–48, https://doi.org/10.1016/j.cpr.2018.06.004.

8. Franco De Crescenzo et al., "Selective Serotonin Reuptake Inhibitors (SSRIs) for Post-Partum Depression (PPD): A Systematic Review of Randomized Clinical Trials," *Journal of Affective Disorders* 152–54 (January 2014): 39–44, https://doi.org/10.1016/j.jad.2013.09.019.

9. Iris Agrawal et al., "Risk Factors of Postpartum Depression," *Cureus* 14, no. 10 (2022): e30898, https://doi.org/10.7759/cureus.30898.

10. Andy Deprato et al., "Impact of Postpartum Physical Activity on Maternal Depression and Anxiety: A Systematic Review and Meta-Analysis," *British Journal of Sports Medicine* 59, no. 8 (2025): 550–61, https://doi.org/10.1136/bjsports-2024-108478.

11. Mi-Mi Zhang et al., "The Efficacy and Safety of Omega-3 Fatty Acids on Depressive Symptoms in Perinatal Women: A Meta-Analysis of Randomized Placebo-Controlled Trials," *Translational Psychiatry* 10, no. 1 (2020): 193, https://doi.org/10.1038/s41398-020-00886-3.

12. Shirin Amini et al., "Postpartum Depression and Vitamin D: A Systematic Review," *Critical Reviews in Food Science and Nutrition* 59, no. 9 (2019): 1514–20, https://doi.org/10.1080/10408398.2017.1423276.

13. Elham Pishevar Hamlbar et al., "The Effect of Curcumin on Postpartum Depression and Anxiety in Primiparous Women: A Double-Blind Randomized Placebo-Controlled Clinical Trial," *BMC Complementary Medicine and Therapies* 25, no. 1 (2025): 157, https://doi.org/10.1186/s12906-025-04798-x.

Edinburgh Postnatal Depression Scale (EPDS)

1. J. L. Cox et al., "Detection of Postnatal Depression: Development of the 10-Item Edinburgh Postnatal Depression Scale," *British Journal of Psychiatry* 150, no. 6 (1987): 782–86, https://doi.org/10.1192/bjp.150.6.782. The form is available online at https://www.sadag.org/images/brochures/edinburghscale.pdf.

Chapter 12 A Different Path to Motherhood

1. "1 in 10 Dads Experience Postpartum Depression, Anxiety: How to Spot the Signs," UT Southwestern Medical Center, August 17, 2021, https://utswmed.org/medblog/paternal-postpartum-depression/.

2. Sarah L. Mott et al., "Depression and Anxiety Among Postpartum and Adoptive Mothers," *Archives of Women's Mental Health* 14, no. 4 (2011): 335–43, https://doi.org/10.1007/s00737-011-0227-1.

3. Karen J. Foli et al., "Post-Adoption Depression: Parental Classes of Depressive Symptoms Across Time," *Journal of Affective Disorders* 200 (August 2016): 293–302, https://doi.org/10.1016/j.jad.2016.01.049.

4. "Chemical Pregnancy," Cleveland Clinic, updated August 14, 2024, https://my.clevelandclinic.org/health/diseases/22188-chemical-pregnancy.

5. "About Stillbirth," US Centers for Disease Control and Prevention, updated August 26, 2025, https://www.cdc.gov/stillbirth/about/index.html.

6. Abigail M. Ramseyer et al., "Cesarean Delivery Management of Stillbirth: In-Depth Analysis of 75 Cases in a Rural State," *South Medical*

Journal 114, no. 7 (2021): 384–87, https://doi.org/10.14423/SMJ.0000000000001267.

7. Ayla Coussa et al., "Impact of Contraception and IVF Hormones on Metabolic, Endocrine, and Inflammatory Status," *Journal of Assisted Reproduction and Genetics* 37, no. 6 (2020): 1267–72, https://doi.org/10.1007/s10815-020-01756-z.

8. Natalie V. Scime et al., "Association Between Infertility and Incident Onset of Systemic Autoimmune Rheumatic Disease after Childbirth: A Population-Based Cohort Study," *Human Reproduction* 40, no. 1 (2025): 157–66, https://doi.org/10.1093/humrep/deae253.

9. Salvatore Gizzo et al., "The Potential Role of GnRH Agonists and Antagonists in Inducing Thyroid Physiopathological Changes During IVF," *Reproductive Sciences* 23, no. 4 (2016): 515–23, https://doi.org/10.1177/1933719115608000.

10. Maria P. Velez et al., "New-Onset Mental Illness Among Gestational Carriers," *JAMA Network Open* 8, no. 7 (2025): e2523428, https://doi.org/10.1001/jamanetworkopen.2025.23428.

11. Karen J. Foli et al., "Rates and Predictors of Depression in Adoptive Mothers: Moving Toward Theory," *Advances in Nursing Science* 35, no. 1 (2012): 51–63, https://doi.org/10.1097/ANS.0b013e318244553e.

12. *Resource Document on Psychiatric Aspects of Infertility* (American Psychiatric Association, 2019), https://www.psychiatry.org/getattachment/51ad144a-20bd-4d6a-bcc6-8f5a163a5f53/Resource-Document-2019-Psychiatric-Aspects-of-Infertility.pdf.

13. Adrian L. Lopresti, "The Effects of Psychological and Environmental Stress on Micronutrient Concentrations in the Body: A Review of the Evidence," *Advances in Nutrition* 11, no. 1 (2020): 103–12, https://doi.org/10.1093/advances/nmz082.

14. Kassem Sharif et al., "The Role of Stress in the Mosaic of Autoimmunity: An Overlooked Association," *Autoimmunity Reviews* 17, no. 10 (2018): 967–83, https://doi.org/10.1016/j.autrev.2018.04.005.

15. Huan Song et al., "Association of Stress-Related Disorders with Subsequent Autoimmune Disease," *JAMA* 319, no. 23 (2018): 2388–400, https://doi.org/10.1001/jama.2018.7028.

16. Christine G. Parks et al., "Life Events, Caregiving, and Risk of Autoimmune Rheumatic Diseases in the Women's Health Initiative Observational Study," *Arthritis Care & Research* 75, no. 12 (2023): 2519–28, https://doi.org/10.1002/acr.25164.

17. Katja Petrowski and George J. Kahaly, "Stress & Thyroid Function—From Bench to Bedside," *Endocrine Reviews* 46, no. 5 (2025), https://doi.org/10.1210/endrev/bnaf015.

18. Mizokami et al., "Stress and Thyroid Autoimmunity," 1047–55.

Chapter 13 A Healthy Postpartum Plan

1. Carlson and Mikes, "Postpartum Thyroiditis."

2. Abigail Perry et al., "Dietary Factors That Affect the Risk of Pre-Eclampsia," *BMJ Nutrition, Prevention & Health* 5, no. 1 (2022): 118–33, https://doi.org/10.1136/bmjnph-2021-000399.

3. Thomas Remer et al., "Short-Term Impact of a Lactovegetarian Diet on Adrenocortical Activity and Adrenal Androgens," *Journal of Clinical Endocrinology & Metabolism* 83, no. 6 (1998): 2132–37, https://doi.org/10.1210/jcem.83.6.4883.

4. Anna-Mariia Shulhai et al., "The Role of Nutrition on Thyroid Function," *Nutrients* 16, no. 15 (2024): 2496, https://doi.org/10.3390/nu16152496.

5. Maryam Ghaedrahmati and Zahra Alipour, "The Association Between Post-Partum Depression and Nutrition and Dietary Patterns: Systematic Review," *Iranian Journal of Nursing and Midwifery Research* 29, no. 3 (2024): 280–89, https://doi.org/10.4103/ijnmr.ijnmr_163_22.

6. Rosaria Maddalena Ruggeri et al., "Nutrition and Autoimmune Diseases," *Nutrients* 17, no. 13 (2025): 2176, https://doi.org/10.3390/nu17132176.

7. Ty Beal and Flaminia Ortenzi, "Priority Micronutrient Density in Foods," *Frontiers in Nutrition* 9 (March 6, 2022), https://doi.org/10.3389/fnut.2022.806566.

8. Beal and Ortenzi, "Priority Micronutrient Density in Foods."

9. Melissa M. Lane et al., "Ultra-Processed Food Exposure and Adverse Health Outcomes: Umbrella Review of Epidemiological Meta-Analyses," *BMJ* (February 28, 2024): 384, https://doi.org/10.1136/bmj-2023-077310.

10. Scott M. Boback et al., "Cooking and Grinding Reduces the Cost of Meat Digestion," *Comparative Biochemistry and Physiology Part A: Molecular & Integrative Physiology* 148, no. 3 (2007): 651–56, https://doi.org/10.1016/j.cbpa.2007.08.014.

11. T. Alan Jiang, "Health Benefits of Culinary Herbs and Spices," *Journal of AOAC International* 102, no. 2 (2019): 395–411, https://doi.org/10.5740/jaoacint.18-0418.

12. D. P. Rose et al., "High-Fiber Diet Reduces Serum Estrogen Concentrations in Premenopausal Women," *American Journal of Clinical Nutrition* 54, no. 3 (1991): 520–25, https://doi.org/10.1093/ajcn/54.3.520.

13. Ghada A. Soliman, "Dietary Fiber, Atherosclerosis, and Cardiovascular Disease," *Nutrients* 11, no. 5 (2019): 1155, https://doi.org/10.3390/nu11051155.

14. Douglas Nitzke et al., "Increasing Dietary Fiber Intake for Type 2 Diabetes Mellitus Management: A Systematic Review," *World Journal of Diabetes* 15, no. 5 (2024): 1001–10, https://doi.org/10.4239/wjd.v15.i5.1001.

15. Zhican Wang et al., "Interplay Between Vitamin D and the Drug Metabolizing Enzyme CYP3A4," *Journal of Steroid Biochemistry and Molecular Biology* 136 (July 2013): 54–58, https://doi.org/10.1016/j.jsbmb.2012.09.012.

16. Christine Blume et al., "Effects of Light on Human Circadian Rhythms, Sleep and Mood," *Somnologie* 23, no. 3 (2019): 147–56, https://doi.org/10.1007/s11818-019-00215-x.

17. Oliver Cameron Reddy and Ysbrand D. van der Werf, "The Sleeping Brain: Harnessing the Power of the Glymphatic System Through Lifestyle Choices," *Brain Sciences* 10, no. 11 (2020): 868, https://doi.org/10.3390/brainsci10110868.

18. Margaret E. Sears et al., "Arsenic, Cadmium, Lead, and Mercury in Sweat: A Systematic Review," *Journal of Environmental and Public Health* (2012): 184745, https://doi.org/10.1155/2012/184745.

19. Kevin P. Madore and Anthony D. Wagner, "Multicosts of Multitasking," *Cerebrum* (April 1, 2019), https://www.ncbi.nlm.nih.gov/pmc/articles/PMC7075496/.

Chapter 14 What About the Good?

1. Karin Modig et al., "Payback Time? Influence of Having Children on Mortality in Old Age," *Journal of Epidemiology and Community Health* 71, no. 5 (2017): 424–30, https://doi.org/10.1136/jech-2016-207857.

2. Leon A. Simons et al., "Childbearing History and Late-Life Mortality: The Dubbo Study of Australian Elderly," *Age and Ageing* 41, no. 4 (2012): 523–28, https://doi.org/10.1093/ageing/afs016.

3. Joanna Orr et al., "Higher Parity Is Associated with Lower Mortality in a European Population of Women with High Fertility: Results From Ireland," *Journal of Gerontology: Series A, Biological Sciences and Medical Sciences* 76, no. 9 (2021): 1571–78, https://doi.org/10.1093/gerona/glaa323.

4. Petra Rattay and Elena von der Lippe, "Association Between Living with Children and the Health and Health Behavior of Women and Men. Are There Differences by Age? Results of the 'German Health Update' (GEDA) Study," *International Journal of Environmental Research and Public Health* 17, no. 9 (2020): 3180, https://doi.org/10.3390/ijerph17093180.

5. Marthe S. Gottschalk et al., "The Relation of Number of Childbirths with Age at Natural Menopause: A Population Study of 310,147 Women in Norway," *Human Reproduction* 37, no. 2 (2022): 333–40, https://doi.org/10.1093/humrep/deab246.

6. Cindy K. Barha et al., "Number of Children and Telomere Length in Women: A Prospective, Longitudinal Evaluation," *PLOS ONE* 11, no. 1 (2016), https://doi.org/10.1371/journal.pone.0146424.

7. Miguel Portela and Paul Schweinzer, "The Parental Co-Immunization Hypothesis: An Observational Competing Risks Analysis," *Scientific Reports* 9, no. 1 (2019): 2493, https://doi.org/10.1038/s41598-019-39124-2.

8. Susan J. Jordan et al., "Pregnancy Outcomes and Risk of Endometrial Cancer: A Pooled Analysis of Individual Participant Data in the Epidemiology of Endometrial Cancer Consortium," *International Journal of Cancer* 148, no. 9 (2021): 2068–78, https://doi.org/10.1002/ijc.33360.

9. Kezia Gaitskell et al., "Histological Subtypes of Ovarian Cancer Associated With Parity and Breastfeeding in the Prospective Million Women Study," *International Journal of Cancer* 142, no. 2 (2018): 281–89, https://doi.org/10.1002/ijc.31063.

10. "Cancer Stat Facts: Common Cancer Sites," National Cancer Institute, accessed September 10, 2025, https://seer.cancer.gov/statfacts/html/common.html.

11. Britta Stordal, "Breastfeeding Reduces the Risk of Breast Cancer: A Call for Action in High-Income Countries with Low Rates of Breastfeeding," *Cancer Medicine* 12, no. 4 (2023): 4616–25, https://doi.org/10.1002/cam4.5288.

12. Stordal, "Breastfeeding Reduces the Risk of Breast Cancer," 4616–25.

13. Portela, "Parental Co-Immunization Hypothesis," 2493.

14. Eva Asselmann et al., "Physical and Mental Health Changes in the Five Years Before and Five Years After Childbirth: A Population-Based Panel Study in First-Time Mothers and Fathers from Germany," *Journal of Affective Disorders* 301 (2022): 138–44, https://doi.org/10.1016/j.jad.2022.01.050.

15. Hanyu Wang et al., "Number of Children and the Prevalence of Later-Life Major Depression and Insomnia in Women and Men: Findings from a Cross-Sectional Study of 0.5 Million Chinese Adults," *BMC Psychiatry* 20, no. 1 (2020): 267, https://doi.org/10.1186/s12888-020-02681-2.

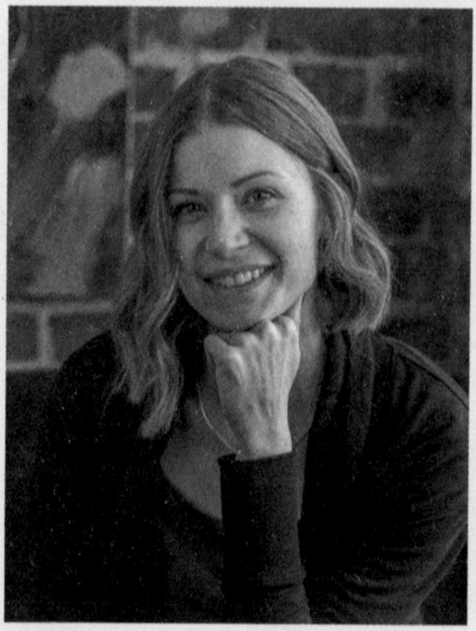

Dr. Alexandra MacKillop is a functional medicine doctor, author, and speaker. Her Substack newsletter focuses on women's health topics, and she sees patients both in person in Chicago and virtually throughout the Midwest. She is also the author of *Fulfilled*, a non-diet book designed to help women repair their relationships with food and their bodies, and *Go with Your Flow*, a functional medicine–focused text on the topic of women's hormones and menstrual health. Dr. MacKillop has two children and lives near Chicago with her family.

Connect with Alexandra:

AlexandraMacKillop.com

INSTAGRAM @DrAlexandraMacKillop